BEFORE I FORGET

BEFORE
I FORGET

LOVE, HOPE, HELP, *and* ACCEPTANCE

in OUR FIGHT AGAINST ALZHEIMER'S

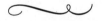

B. SMITH & DAN GASBY

With Michael Shnayerson

FOREWORD BY RUDOLPH E. TANZI, PHD

HARMONY

BOOKS • NEW YORK

Published in the United States by Harmony Books, an imprint of the Crown Publishing
Group, a division of Penguin Random House LLC, New York.
www.crownpublishing.com

Harmony Books is a registered trademark, and the Circle colophon is a trademark of
Penguin Random House LLC.

Library of Congress Cataloging-in-Publication Data
Smith, B. (Barbara), 1949–
Before I forget / B. Smith and Dan Gasby.—First edition.
pages cm
1. Smith, B. (Barbara), 1949–   2. Gasby, Dan.   3. Alzheimer's disease—Biography.
4. Husband and wife—Biography.   5. Alzheimer's disease—Family relationships.
I. Gasby, Dan.
RC523.2.S634 2015
616.8'310092—dc23
[B]   2015009839

ISBN 978-0-553-44712-5
eBook ISBN 978-0-553-44713-2

Printed in the United States of America

Book design by Amanda Dewey
Jacket design by Jess Morphew
Jacket photography by Heather Weston

10 9 8 7 6 5 4 3 2 1

First Edition

To the men and women of the U.S. Congress who have the power to help spare future generations from the ravages of Alzheimer's . . . and to all who will be helped by them.

Contents

FOREWORD

by Rudolph E. Tanzi, PhD

It haunts us with every name we forget: the fear that Alzheimer's is in our future.

For many of us, those lapses will be nothing more than the natural aging process. But for an estimated 5.2 million Americans, Alzheimer's has taken hold—and to most of us in the field, that number is way too low. Millions more die of Alzheimer's-provoked causes, from organ failure to pneumonia. Alzheimer's is a thief that robs you of your memories, your personality, ultimately of your self. It pulls apart the tapestry of who you are thread by thread, until the tapestry just disappears. Cancer is the Big C, but many now overcome it. With the Big A, to date, not one person has survived.

In one sense, we have modern medicine to blame. At the dawn of the twentieth century, our lifespan was forty-nine years. Most of our forebears who carried Alzheimer's-linked genes didn't live long enough to develop the disease. Now many of us live into our eighties: by eighty-five, a third will have Alzheimer's and half will be in the earliest stages of the disease. Nearly 75 million baby boomers are heading that way. Already, Medicare and Medicaid are staggering under the costs. I calculate that by 2020, if the federal government fails to take drastic measures, they may reach a tipping point and start to collapse.

Each year, the federal government spends $6–12 billion on each of the usual suspects: cancer, heart disease, and AIDS. It spends less than $500 million on Alzheimer's. Of that, perhaps only $250 million goes to basic research; much of the rest goes to carrying out large-scale clinical trials for drugs that have, so far, without exception, failed. In his 2015 State of the Union speech, President Obama pledged another $50 million for Alzheimer's. Unfortunately, it's a Band-Aid on a gaping wound.

Why the shocking lack of funding? One reason is that the young tend to protest more loudly and actively than their parents and grandparents. And of those who have Alzheimer's, how many are likely to be lobbying in Washington about the loss of their minds? But as I warned last year's graduating class at the University of Rhode Island, the young may want to reconsider their lack of interest in Alzheimer's—for almost entirely selfish reasons.

Those graduates will likely live to be eighty-five or ninety years old, if not one hundred. That means more of them—far more—will get Alzheimer's than cancer or heart disease. They may see it as their aging grandparents' problem. In the long run, it's *theirs*. Not only that: they have parents. By their fifties, many of those graduates will hope to have put their own children through college and be spending those later decades traveling the world. No way: not with parents succumbing to Alzheimer's. Through gritted teeth, those graduates will be spending their savings on assisted care and nursing homes and hospice care. Even now, Alzheimer's is not just a disease of the old. It affects us all, and will do so more deeply within the next decade.

Here's the good news. Alzheimer's is probably the most striking example we have among major diseases of a budget-constrained problem. As opposed, that is, to a knowledge-constrained one. We know what we need to do. We have dozens of gene candidates to work on, each one of which can present a new opportunity for drug development. We just lack the money to do that work.

The bad news is that Alzheimer's isn't merely under-represented in funding compared with those other diseases. Those genes we need to look at? Together, we in the field have less than 5 percent of the funding we need to pursue their potential. I'm more fortunate than most; I've published nearly five hundred research papers, and my lab gets serious attention from the National Institutes of Health. Younger scientists in less well-known labs struggle for even the most essential funds to continue. There's so little money in science and research in the United States that more and more students choose not to enter the field. The result: our country faces losing a generation or two of scientists, and all the work they would do. If America does not step up and start funding medical research more seriously, we will rapidly lose our place as a world leader in biomedical discovery. While pharmaceutical companies are needed to bring drugs to the market, the seeds of discovery begin in academic institutions, which depend on federal funding to survive. I am also lucky to be funded by the Cure Alzheimer's Fund (http://curealz.org), the most forward-thinking and -looking Alzheimer's research foundation in the world, in my opinion.

Yes, we do at last know which way to proceed. After decades of debate about how Alzheimer's forms in the human brain, we know what the pathologies are, and how they progress, along with the genes that are responsible. Those genes provoke the creation of amyloid plaques. The plaques then cause so-called tau tangles to form in the surrounding brain cells, eventually to kill those cells. Plaques also cause inflammation, which kills more cells, leading to even more inflammation in a vicious cycle. As our "Alzheimer's-in-a-Dish" studies have shown, the amyloid sets the fire, if you will, and tangles are the fire that spreads throughout the brain; inflammation fans the flames and makes the fire spread that much faster.

Here's something else we know now: the amyloid plaques start building up in the brain at least fifteen years before the disease manifests itself. So we know we have to detect plaques far sooner. Then we must have therapies ready to slow them down, akin to lowering cholesterol, if it is too high, to prevent heart disease.

Nearly all of us will develop at least a few of those plaques, though not all of us will get Alzheimer's. Why? More and more, we think inflammation is key. While plaques and tangles may push you up the mountain, it is inflammation that throws you off the cliff. In the process of inflammation, certain immune cells in your brain kill nerve cells in response to the pathology, leading to a massive loss of nerve cells and the neural circuitry needed for learning and memory.

So we have three mantras going forward: early prediction, early detection, and then early prevention. We will use genetics to predict risk, biomarkers and imaging to detect the disease before symptoms, and then steps to prevent the disease from taking root in those with the strongest propensity to develop it.

We need the right drug, but we also need the right patient— not every one may respond equally to one drug or another.

And we need to know how soon to administer that drug when we do get it. In my lab, we're working on two drugs that seem extremely promising in terms of stopping plaque and tangle growth early on. We are also searching for drugs that will stop the inflammation from spreading. We are lucky to be working with exciting new genetic data about inflammation, obtained from the Alzheimer's Genome Project, also supported by the Cure Alzheimer's Fund.

I wish fervently that I could say to B. Smith and her husband, Dan, that these drugs will reach the market soon enough to keep B.'s Alzheimer's from progressing. I can't. The truth is that at this rate, given the funding we have, our plaque/tangle drug will need another decade in development, the inflammation drug a bit longer than that. If we threw billions more at our research efforts, we could cut that time frame by years. But that's not likely to happen.

For those who have Alzheimer's now, there are lifestyle measures that may allay some symptoms of the disease—measures that B. and Dan report on in this helpful and poignant book. There is also so much that family caregivers can learn about how to deal with Alzheimer's: its many emotional challenges, its hardships, and, if one is looking, the state of grace it sometimes brings.

Alzheimer's is a hard, hard diagnosis to cope with, and I have enormous empathy with those who are doing it. Perhaps it will seem of little comfort to them, but the fact is, I have never been more optimistic about the prospect of treating this disease. It will take time—too much time. Heartbreaking time. But we will get there. Of that, I have no doubt.

PART I

LITTLE SIGNS OF
DIFFERENCE

I know where I'm going. I'm still myself. I just can't remember things as well as I once did. So on short trips, I work hard not to be confused. I'll say to myself, "What are we going to do? How long are we staying?" It's like I'm talking to my other self— the self I used to be. She tells me, "This is what we need to buy— not that." I'm conscious of that other self guiding me now.

Here at the house I'm fine. Sometimes it takes me a little longer to get dressed than it used to; sometimes I forget what I put on the stove. But that's just normal, right?

Actually, I know it's not just normal. I know I have Alzheimer's. I know I have to work harder than before to keep things straight and do what Dan says. So I do! It doesn't always work out, though, and Dan gets frustrated with me. I get frustrated with him, too. We're both very strong people, in our own different ways— I'm quieter, he's not—and both of us speak our minds.

The thing is, before all this happened, we never argued. A little grumble here or there but that was it. Everything just went like a breeze. And we had fun! We had a lot of fun together, every day, coming up with new ideas, making them work. That seems a long time ago now.

Lately, I've been wanting to go home. Not the house that Dan *and I have here, wonderful as it is, but home, to Everson, Pennsylvania, where I grew up. It's been such a while since I was there. Dan doesn't want me to drive there, and so I won't misbehave and drive without him knowing it—although I'd like to! I'll let him drive. Maybe this time I'll take my parents down with me.*

No—I don't mean that. Just saying that aloud reminds me they're no longer alive. I do have a problem remembering that. That's the only thing that bothers me. I don't know why, but it does. I guess because every time I forget and remember, it's like going through mourning again, with that same pang you felt in the pit of your stomach the first time you heard that your mother or father died. I feel that pang every time I remember.

ONE

SAG HARBOR

June 2014

We are blessed in many ways, not the least of which is by the view we wake to every day now: the wide blue bay between Sag Harbor and Shelter Island, in that part of the world they call the Hamptons, at the east end of Long Island, New York. Our house is on the beach, perfect for early morning walks. We used to take those walks together. Now I head down on my own while Barbara sleeps in, her body clock submerged like some treasure at the bottom of the bay.

By 9 a.m., I can hear Barbara rustling around in her clothes closet, looking for something to wear. The closet is crammed full, which drives me crazy. Barbara refuses to go through her wardrobe and give to Goodwill the outfits she's not worn for years. She won't let me in there to help her, either. That closet is her domain. "So let's get someone else to come in and organize you," I say. "Someone whose judgment you trust, who can go through your closet and organize it with you."

"Like who?"

"Like . . . I don't know. Someone."

"I don't want fashion help."

And so the closet stays as it is, and Barbara emerges from it, dressed at last. Sometimes she looks as put together as when I first met her, a quarter century ago: B. Smith, international fashion model and lifestyle guru, publishing and television star, a national brand. A woman who on any given day changed outfits three times for three different public venues—a woman so fashion-savvy she knew how to tie my ties backward on me.

Then there are mornings like this one, when B. comes out in a Christmas sweater, corduroys, and black boots.

"You can't wear that, sweetie," I tell her gently. "Those clothes are for winter, and we're here in June."

Barbara's first reaction is a flash of anger—an emotion I rarely saw before all this started. The anger gives way to tears she wipes with her hand. She never used to cry, either. B. was the happiest woman I ever knew. Also, the most beautiful.

She's still the most beautiful.

Hanging her head, B. goes back to her closet to try again while I make the tea and a healthy breakfast: fresh-squeezed grapefruit juice, berries, and bananas. We used to have toast, too, or muffins or scones. They're gone from our diet now: no bread in this house. No carbohydrates of any kind: no potatoes, no rice, no pasta. No fatty dairy foods like cheese and butter. No red meat, either—except bison burgers, which are really lean meat and satisfy our occasional yen for a juicy hamburger. Chicken—organically grown—is okay. Just no processed chicken or meat of any kind. Mostly, a Mediterranean diet is what we go by these days. Seasonal fruits for breakfast, fresh vegetables for lunch and dinner, cooked in olive oil or, even better, grapeseed oil, briefly and on high heat to retain their flavor and nutritional value. A lot of fish, but not large fish that have high concentrations of mercury; instead cold-water fish like fluke, flounder, freshwater salmon, and cod. The smaller the fish, the better: a superhealthy choice is sardines. All these are rich in omega-3 fatty acids, good for the heart—and the brain.

We eat breakfast looking out on the bay. Barbara's second try at an outfit for the day is better—weather appropriate, at least. If it weren't, I don't think I could bear to tell her so.

Before all this happened, we'd tell each other our plans for the day. Barbara might have a meeting with her editor about her next lifestyle and entertaining book. Or a photo shoot for one of the products she represented. Or a design session with Bed Bath & Beyond about some of the four hundred licensed B. Smith home products the chain carries, everything from sheets and towels to perfume to bath oils. I took care of business— B.'s business, which was our business. I had my hands full with licensee deals, pitching new television food shows, and finding new ways to extend the brand. I had a whole other job managing our three B. Smith restaurants—in Manhattan, Sag Harbor, and Washington, D.C. It was a lot of work, but there was a sense of momentum; the B. Smith brand was growing. There was a lot to talk about. Now there's less. I've had to cut back on meetings and plans to take care of B. Most of the business I do is on phone calls stolen from caregiver time.

So my plans, this morning, are loose. As for B., she has no plans today. She sits there at the breakfast table, the love of my life, waiting quietly for me to tell her what to do.

I used to look at those couples in restaurants that never talk—you know the ones I mean. How could they stay together?

Thank God we weren't like that! We still aren't—not in the sense I meant when I looked at those other couples. We still love each other—a lot. But there's much more quiet time now. I'm the one who has to initiate conversation. Barbara understands what I'm saying, and will answer readily enough. But after a sentence or two, she'll peter out. She doesn't know how to get from sentence A to sentence C or D, so after a moment, she lapses into silence. She also may not remember, five minutes later, what it was we talked about.

So I come up with plans of a sort for B. Walk the dog. Drive with me into Sag Harbor. Shop for dinner. She can do all those tasks when I'm with her. Some she can still do on her own—so far. But we have to tackle those plans right away. We can't say we'll do them in an hour or two. If we do, they'll swirl out of Barbara's mind like so many grains of sand swept down the beach. Then, after that hour or two, I'll have to repeat the plans, and tell her it's time to go. She'll perk up, nod at this new information, and give me that heartbreaking smile.

Time is elastic for Barbara—that's the word I use. A moment stretches to infinity; a day shrinks to no time at all. In public, she is as poised as ever. At the American Hotel (one of my favorites), she greets strangers warmly, makes small talk, and laughs. She did that so naturally at her own restaurants that she does it whenever we go out. Perhaps a few of our fellow diners find this a bit odd; most are delighted. They know Barbara from television, books, and restaurants, or just from her presence around town.

In a funny way, Alzheimer's is perfect for celebrities. They greet people without being expected to know who those people are. They have brief, happy chats about nothing in particular.

And then they move on, before anyone figures out that for people with Alzheimer's, the small talk just gets smaller and smaller.

The painful truth is that the woman who's greeting them so warmly has no idea what day of the week it is.

She has no idea what year it is, either.

TWO

SAG HARBOR

June 2014

About nine months ago, when B. was diagnosed, I learned the numbers. Some 5.2 million Americans are living with Alzheimer's. About 500,000 of those die of the disease each year, even as more than that get diagnosed: a new case every sixty-seven seconds. It used to be the sixth leading cause of death in the United States. Last year one study moved it up to third, just behind heart disease and cancer. Why? Because all too often, the researchers noted, a patient dies of an illness or condition that Alzheimer's produces—like pneumonia, or organ failure—and doctors list that as the cause of death. If instead they listed Alzheimer's in those cases—the root cause—the total would go way up, putting Alzheimer's above chronic lung disease, stroke, and accidents. Way to go, right? That would mean *millions* die of it every year. But however you want to define the death toll, one in nine Americans age sixty-five or older has it: 11 percent of the senior population. That shoots up to 33 percent for all Americans eighty-five and older.

The number that really rocked me was this one: 200,000. That's how many Americans under sixty-five have Alzheimer's. They call it early-onset Alzheimer's, as opposed to late-onset, which is everyone sixty-five and older. Early-onset is a genetic disease; late-onset is, too, but it's complicated by lifestyle choices and aging.

I thought about that number a lot. My first reaction was anger and incredulity. In this whole country, only 200,000 people under sixty-five have early-onset Alzheimer's, and B. gets targeted as one of them? How unfair is that? Who's the manager in charge here? I want to talk to him *right now*.

Then I thought: wow, 200,000. That's a lot of people. Imagine them all in one place, milling around together. Like Woodstock. Actually a lot of today's 200,000 probably *were* at Woodstock. They're just as spaced-out now as they were then.

That's what passes for humor in the world of Alzheimer's. And let me tell you one dead serious thing I've learned about that: whatever humor you can find here, no matter how off-color or corny—or raunchy—you take it. You need all the laughter you can get. A stupid joke won't change the picture, but it might enliven a moment, and that's where people with Alzheimer's— and their caregivers—live. In the moment. So laugh if you can, at any excuse. Even if that moment is soon forgotten, replaced by the next.

Two hundred thousand. Imagine that. Two hundred thousand households where a family member under sixty-five wakes in a fog every morning, as B. does, and drifts through the day needing constant guidance from a loved one or hired caregiver. Yet that's just a sliver of the overall Alzheimer's population.

Here's another number that blew me away. Of those 5.2

million Americans with Alzheimer's, two-thirds are women. A
woman of sixty-five has a 1-in-6 chance of getting Alzheimer's
at some point in her remaining years—versus a man's 1-in-11
chance. The difference is in part because women tend to live
longer, and the aging process seems to exacerbate the genetic
and lifestyle factors associated with the disease.

Even more surprising than the high incidence of women getting Alzheimer's is this: African Americans are twice as likely as
Caucasians to get it. Ten percent over sixty-five have it. By the age
of eighty-five, *half* of all African Americans have it. Why that's
so is one of the many mysteries of this insidious disease. Genetic risk factors seem to be involved. Diabetes, with its higher
incidence in the black community, seems to increase susceptibility. So do hypertension and cardiovascular disease. But African
Americans, it turns out, also tend to ignore the symptoms of Alzheimer's longer than whites, either viewing them as part of the
aging process or not wanting to learn what they fear and suspect
is true. There's a stigma to Alzheimer's—a terrible stigma, greater
than that for most diseases—and African Americans seem to feel
it even more keenly than whites. So they often take their fears to
a doctor years later than they should, too late for the changes in
diet and exercise that might help stave off the symptoms.

B. has lived in the public eye for a long time, from her first
days as a black fashion model in an all-white industry to
her rise as B. Smith, restaurateur, cookbook writer, magazine
publisher, and television food and style maven. For all the challenges we face with Alzheimer's, one choice was easily made,
almost as soon as B. got diagnosed. B. would live this part of her

life in the public eye, too, as a spokesperson for all Americans struggling with Alzheimer's, but especially for women, even more so women of color. From our first conversation about it, B. has never wavered from that intent, nor have I.

By telling her story here, B. might help others recognize the symptoms of Alzheimer's sooner—and take action sooner. We knew all too well how mystifying and maddening those symptoms could be before we learned what they were. For more than a year, our marriage had been shaken by flare-ups and hurt feelings we'd never experienced before. We were the kind of couple that finished each other's sentences, happy together all day and night—which, as partners in business as in life, we were. Suddenly we were arguing—over B.'s forgetfulness, and my anger in response. Raising voices, scoring points, slamming doors. I had begun to wonder if love had left the room. Maybe this marriage of nearly twenty years was coming to an end. Knowing that B. had the first symptoms of Alzheimer's wouldn't have done a thing to keep the disease from worsening as it did. But it would have given us another year, maybe two, of the old normal—or at least some semblance of it—and helped us cope with the memory lapses, and mood swings, when they occurred.

That was one reason for B. to go public. Another was to motivate African Americans to put the stigma of Alzheimer's aside and get involved in a crucial way. For decades, too few of us have volunteered for research and clinical trials, so scientists have been kept from figuring out why we do get Alzheimer's more often than whites. Without a representative sampling of African Americans in those trials, scientists can't be sure that the drugs they're trying to develop for the disease work as well—or at all—with us. There are reasons, historically, for being wary of those trials, but the truth is we're hurting our people by not participating at this point. If we want our children and grand-children not to have Alzheimer's, more of us have to participate in those trials.

There was one more critical reason for B. and me to get out there. Finding and testing new drugs is expensive. Like $1 billion for each next candidate. We all know that drug companies make big profits when they come up with a winner. But those drugs save lives. So far with Alzheimer's, and unfortunately for all of us, they haven't come up with any winners. They've lost tens of billions of dollars trying to deal with the disease—not even to cure it, just to keep it in check. They've basically come up dry. Like it or not, the federal government has to do more than it's doing: spend more taxpayer dollars helping the drug companies come up with the magic bullet. That means taxpay-ers pushing to see their money get spent that way.

By telling our story, B. and I have joined a campaign of doc-tors, scientists, and policy makers, among others, who see 2020 as the target date for managing Alzheimer's and are doing all they can to hit that target. Not for curing it, not for preventing it—not yet for either of those. Just for catching it earlier, and maybe—maybe—keeping it in check so that patients live longer and keep some semblance of the lives they had before this awful disease afflicted them.

Since her diagnosis, by the way, I'm pleased to report that B.'s status has changed. She's no longer one of those 200,000 early-onset victims of Alzheimer's.

She's turned sixty-five.

THREE

SAG HARBOR

July 2014

Some doctors see Alzheimer's as a disease of seven stages. Others see it as a three-stage disease. It's the same disease either way: it doesn't progress any slower if you measure it in seven stages rather than three. Whichever model you use, B. has the mildest stage. That's what her doctors told her last autumn when she was diagnosed. Her short-term memory is diminished, but her long-term memory, so far, is fine. She needs my help in an ongoing way—so far, I'm her one and only caregiver—but she still gets around on her own, at least from our house into town. She drives to the market, picks up the mail—all the daily errands that anyone in a small town does on her own.

I know that at some point, she won't be able to drive anymore, and I know she won't be the one to decide that. I will. I also know that she'll be angry—really angry—when I cut her off and start keeping the keys in some secret place. I can live with that, and the anger, after all, will pass. It always does, along with the hurt. What bothers me is: How will I know when that time has come? When she gets lost coming home? When she gets into an accident? When either she, or someone else, is hurt? I know the right thing would be to take the keys from her now. But I also know how that would depress her, robbing her of her independence and making her feel worse than she does. I try to keep B. as happy as I can, while also trying to keep her safe.

Almost every afternoon, B. takes Bishop, our Italian mastiff, for a walk on the beach. Those are some of her happiest times. Bishop came into our lives after B. was diagnosed: he belonged to our twenty-seven-year-old daughter, Dana, who moved from Washington, D.C., to help, and brought Bishop with her. He's a big and powerful creature who would chomp your arm off if you made a lunge for any one of us. If you'd asked B. or me two years ago what kind of dog we might like, Italian mastiff wouldn't have been on the list. It would now. Bishop is smart; we really communicate. More important, I know that B. will be safe whenever he's with her. I'm not sure B. can sense danger anymore—not from someone who might at first be friendly. But Bishop can.

We live in a neighborhood of Sag Harbor called Sag Harbor Hills—one of three beachfront black communities, side by side. Back in the 1940s, black doctors and lawyers brought their families to this all-but-deserted bayside stretch of scrub pines and sand on the outskirts of what was then a scruffy blue-collar town. The roads were dirt, and pitch dark at night: no streetlights till the 1980s. There these mostly upper-middle-class families summered with their own, rarely renovating or expanding their beachy bungalows. Living below their means was the whole idea, like summer camp. Once in the 1980s, feminist Betty Friedan, novelist E. L. Doctorow, and others tried to bridge the gap between black and white with what they called the Sag Harbor Initiative. It was well intended, but went nowhere; neither side had much interest in socializing with the other. Those three little enclaves—Sag Harbor Hills, Azurest, and Ninevah—are still a draw for prosperous blacks, like Oak Bluffs on Martha's Vineyard, and you're as likely to see Ivy League sweatshirts there as you do in the nearly all-white historic district of Sag Harbor itself. Now, though, the real estate market is bringing integration after all, as black owners die off and white buyers move in, eager to get a waterfront house at a fraction of what it would cost anywhere else in Sag Harbor. A lot of our neighbors resent the changes. Not B. or me. We've always been comfortable in either camp—which is, to be honest, one reason we've done as well as we have. B. just radiates warmth and elegance and grace in a way that transcends race altogether. It's an amazing thing to see—even now.

From our house, B. takes Bishop up the beach toward town, throwing a tennis ball into the surf again and again, and laughing as Bishop swims out to retrieve it. From our front deck, I watch her playing with him, as if nothing were wrong and this day was a day like all the others we've had. Then slowly, steadily, she diminishes, until she's a distant dot.

If she keeps on into town, B. will reach the wharf, and the restaurant that was, until last year, B. Smith's, with its waterfront tables overlooking the marina. For sixteen years we made it a go-to place for whites *and* blacks. To find another such place, where both worlds overlapped, you'd have to go all the way to Manhattan—to the B. Smith's on West Forty-Sixth Street. The B. Smith's in Sag Harbor was also the only black-owned business greater than family-sized in the Hamptons, clear up to Montauk.

B. knows better than to pass the restaurant directly on her walks. She knows that seeing it as someone else's place will make her sad. I think she knows, too, that it would still be hers if not for Alzheimer's. Instead, she turns up Main Street, with Bishop pulling at his leash, and takes in Sag Harbor's simple delights, chatting with other strollers, and perhaps picking up a head of lettuce at the IGA before heading back home—the home that so far she knows how to find.

FOUR

New York City

Fall 2010–Fall 2012

It started four years ago, maybe five, though I can't say for sure, since it crept up so quietly, with just a little thing here or there that didn't seem right. I'm superclean, and B. is, too, and yet she started leaving things around, both at our Sag Harbor house and our Manhattan apartment: a cup, a plate, a can of juice. I started noting that food was left in the fridge until it went bad. We're in the restaurant business; we know not to do that. Often it was because she'd bought not just one container of milk but four or five. *What's with all the milk?* I'd ask her. She'd just shrug.

At first B. didn't appear to have memory lapses. She just seemed thoughtless. One day she took my wallet, put it on top of the car, and drove off. I searched at least half a mile up the road, but never found it. In it, along with my license and credit cards, was a US Medal of Honor coin from a friend who'd had his hand blown off by a grenade in Afghanistan in 2008 yet had gone on to save other soldiers under fire. Over the years in our restaurants, B. and I had hosted several receptions for US

Congressional Medal of Honor winners in conjunction with the USO, and we'd become known for that in the veterans' community. Leroy Petry, the victim of that grenade, had come up to me at the bar of our Manhattan restaurant and said, "I want to give you a hand for all you've done for veterans," then he took off his hand—his prosthetic hand—and gave it to me! It was a joke but one hell of a moment. Leroy took his hand back but then gave me his Medal of Honor coin—for keeps. I was livid at losing that coin.

Then there was the day B. left the roof open on our Mercedes-Benz G-Wagen. That night we had a three-inch rainstorm. I went out the next morning to find the truck looking like an aquarium. Later, I would take to calling it our WTF period, as in *What the fuck?!* There's a song I like by the O'Jays called "Little Signs of Difference." That's what I started to see.

Our daughter Dana was the one who first noticed that B. was repeating herself. Down in D.C., Dana had a long phone conversation with her. An hour later, B. called and launched into the same conversation again. Dana heard her out without letting on. She tried to look at the bright side. B. was still functioning, still cooking and taking care of herself. Most important, she was still making her nightly rounds at our restaurants in Manhattan or Sag Harbor, chatting easily with the customers. Maybe she was just worn down. It was like a storm, Dana thought, a storm that would surely pass.

When was that first time, the first sign? For some reason, that haunted me later—not knowing, or not remembering, that first red flag. There must have been a day when B.

asked me a question, and then an hour or so later asked it again, and I, in my happy, work-focused life, stayed oblivious to what the message really was. I know it was a first shout from B.'s brain, but I still think of it as something outside our world of two, finding its way in, like a fog coming under the door.

By the summer of 2013, though, it was impossible to miss. *Something* was going on. Along with the memory lapses, I noticed the emotional ups and downs. When I spoke with her, B. would seem preoccupied, unresponsive. Finally I'd say, "What's wrong with you?" But that only made her withdraw more. If I kept insisting she say what was really on her mind, she'd burst out with "I hate you! I love you, but I hate you."

B. was the kindest person I'd ever known—kinder even than my own mother. Yet now she might snap at small things, leaving me hurt and confused. And to tell the truth, I would snap back.

It wears on you. Suddenly I was in this bizarre world where B. might be nice and loving one minute, then explode the next. We had been together more than twenty years. We'd never experienced explosions like that.

As the hurt reverberated, I wondered if B. was having an affair. Was it possible? No. I *knew* B. That simply wasn't in her emotional makeup. But then, neither were these flare-ups.

I had always been a night owl, which in the restaurant business counts as a plus. I loved holding forth at our bar, making customers feel at home. To be honest, if those customers were women, all the better. I loved my wife; I'd never cheated on her, nor would I. We were together for life. But I did like flirting. And with B.'s latest accusations ringing in my ears, getting some positive reinforcement from regulars at the bar was all the sweeter. After all, I was just doing my job, was I not?

Yes, I was—while my marriage was teetering on the brink.

For all the numbers we have on Alzheimer's, here's one we don't have: how many marriages end each year amid bitter arguments between couples who think their love has departed, when in fact Alzheimer's has arrived. Couples start to feel out of synch. Our marriage was one of them, for at least a year, as the arguments worsened with nothing other than normal-seeming forgetfulness to accompany them. I'm not proud of this now, but the fact is I started spending more evenings out, not just at our restaurant's bar but at others. Often I walked home late at night through the streets of the city, wondering if our marriage was ending and a new and painful chapter was about to begin.

The turbulence we felt wasn't just shaking our home. Neither B. nor I had ever been late to meetings. Now we were. I would tell B. she was due somewhere at 3 p.m.—as her business manager, I set up her meetings for her—and put it out of my mind as I went off somewhere else. The call would come at 3:15 p.m.: Where was she? I would have to make apologies, go back to the apartment, and get her down there or go myself instead. God forbid they should be morning meetings. B. had always awakened early and jumped into her day. Now if I was gone for the morning, she might just stay asleep. The dynamo I'd married was meandering through her days like a lazy river.

There was more. If B. addressed an audience, she might start with the written remarks before her, then start talking off the cuff—not a bad thing for a public speaker to do, but that wasn't B. She had always given her talks as carefully planned, especially on television. I called her "One-Take B." For eight years, filming her nationally syndicated TV show *B. Smith with Style,* she'd nailed every segment the first time. The director might ask for three or four more takes, just to be sure, but he would end up shaking his head in amazement: the first take was always the best. Now she needed to do multiple takes for a taped television spot, and despite her radiant smile when the camera rolled, there was hesitancy in how she spoke and even how she moved.

That was when she started asking me the same question more than once. Then more than twice. The thought of Alzheimer's never crossed my mind. B. was a very vital sixty-two years old. I'd noticed my own memory slipping somewhat: names, for the most part. Surely that was happening to B., too, just at a slightly faster rate. So I kept making excuses for her.

The next red flag went up in New Orleans. We were down there on business, staying in a nice hotel, and had just spent a wonderful evening in the French Quarter. B. had had her lapses that day, but nothing big enough to get on my nerves and provoke an argument. After a great dinner of jambalaya and crawfish étouffée at Commander's Palace, washed down with some good red wine, we fell into bed. I woke up to someone pounding on the door. The first thing I noticed was that B. wasn't in bed beside me. I opened the door to find her, in her pajamas and bathrobe, between two security guards.

She had been sleepwalking.

Still, the word *Alzheimer's* never entered my mind. What was an incident of sleepwalking in a strange place but normal disorientation? Looking back, I know I had entered that strange, shadowy country they call Denial. It's the first of those five stages of dealing with, and ultimately accepting, loss, whether in regard to life or love; I guess those stages probably apply, in about the same order, to accepting a loved one's diagnosis of Alzheimer's. We had no diagnosis yet, so I did what all deniers do: looked for any other explanation than the one staring me in the face.

Then came the morning we couldn't shrug off: the morning all of us saw B. needed help.

B. had a guest spot on the *Today* show to demonstrate recipes for a Labor Day picnic: chili-spiced chicken wings and jerk shrimp with mixed fruit.

She had done *Today* many times. She felt totally at ease with the whole on-air cast, and the crew loved her, too; the stagehands and directors always greeted her like family. There was, of course, always that moment before she went on: a little twinge of awareness that this was live television. Anything can happen. Focus! But for B., that's all it was: she really loved live TV. Which was also to say, she really loved talking to people.

As I watched from the green room, I saw B. take her place at the food table and slip happily into conversation with co-hosts Peter Alexander and Savannah Guthrie. Then it was as if B. stopped hearing what they were saying. One of them asked her a question. Instead of answering, she just kind of went blank. Ten seconds is an eternity on live television; B. stood there for longer than that.

I stood up in that empty room, horrified as I looked at the screen. Memory lapses—okay, sure. But B. was a pro. She knew the first rule of live television: *fill the space.* If you don't know the answer, say something else; they can't go back and ask it again. Tell them how your mother made buffalo wings and boiled shrimp when you were a girl. Tell about how you just went to New Orleans and had chicken and shrimps there. But no—nothing. Just the deafening sound of television silence. Finally Savannah and Peter started talking to each other as B. nodded and smiled, and the spot concluded at last.

Usually when B. came backstage after an appearance, I'd high-five her and give her a hug. Not this time. I just couldn't fake it.

"Not so good?" B. asked meekly.

"Not so good," I replied.

That was the day both of us had to admit that something was terribly wrong, and that we would have to seek medical help. In retrospect, it was the end of B.'s life as a healthy, happy woman—wife, stepmother, entrepreneur—and the start of a new life, as a person with Alzheimer's.

It was, of course, the end of one life and the start of another for me, too, not just as B.'s partner in marriage and business, but in a role I had never expected to play: her full-time caregiver.

Neither of us had any idea how challenging it would be.

LESSONS LEARNED

Every family's struggle with Alzheimer's is different, every set of circumstances unique. Yet the basic progression of the disease is all too similar from case to case. While nothing can yet be done to modify or arrest the course of Alzheimer's, the symptoms that B. began to experience at age sixty-two can sometimes be offset, at least to a degree, with commonsense measures and compassion. Here are a few suggestions for how to deal with those symptoms and maximize brain health—suggestions that we learned from our own experiences, backed by a lot of reading of other books about Alzheimer's. Our hope is that our own hard-earned wisdom may be of help to you in your own situation.

Before we go there, we ought to be sure we're all on the same page for what we're dealing with here. What is Alzheimer's, and what causes it? Simply put, it's a disease that kills brain cells. The cells it kills first govern memory, especially short-term memory, and so memory loss is usually the first indication that someone is afflicted with the disease. As it progresses, an afflicted person's long-term memory diminishes, too. Eventually, Alzheimer's affects those parts of the brain that control actions and processes we take for granted, from the five senses to physical coordination to swallowing to continence. It is, unfortunately, both progressive and, so far, irreversible.

What causes Alzheimer's? Scientists have plenty of clues, but not the whole progression yet. They know that genes play a part—and when someone as young as B. gets Alzheimer's, scientists go so far as to say that genes are the whole story. Just which genes, exactly, and in what interactions, they continue to debate. But for early-onset Alzheimer's, as they call it in these cases where a person is under sixty-five years old, they feel confident that defective genes are the cause.

With older patients, genes almost certainly play a part, too, but so do a lot of environmental factors, from poor diet and lack of exercise to various aspects of aging. More on them later.

DRESSING INAPPROPRIATELY

My daily challenge of getting B. dressed in appropriate clothing is an all-too-common drama in Alzheimer's households. So, too, is the piling up of clothes in the closet. Early on, I would react by asking—then demanding—that B. clean out her closet. That, as I was forced to concede, was not the right approach. It didn't work. B. insisted that every last item of clothing remain, and in no uncertain terms barred me from the closet!

In retrospect, I realize I might have tried making a series of nocturnal raids on the closet—not cleaning out large piles of old clothing at once, just a few old sweaters and shirts at a time. To avoid any risk of discovery, I might have stored them for a while to see if B. remembered them. If she didn't, I could then donate them to charity. By gradually adding clothes of just one or two basic colors, I could simplify her wardrobe over time so that whatever outfit B. chose would be coordinated.

This is, of course, easier to do with a patient who isn't as fashion-conscious as B.!

THE MEDITERRANEAN DIET

After decades of dismissing any link between diet and Alzheimer's, conventional wisdom has now changed to accept at

least the possibility that a diet rich in omega-3 fatty acids—the
so-called Mediterranean diet—can help alleviate cognitive decline with Alzheimer's patients.

One game-changer was a 2010 report in the *Journal of Alzheimer's Disease* with the catchy title "Effectiveness of the
Mediterranean Diet: Can It Help Delay or Prevent Alzheimer's Disease?" Working with a large study group, the authors
concluded that "a greater adherence to Mediterranean diet
[showed] a reduced risk of major chronic degenerative diseases,
including Alzheimer's." A 2013 study with 17,000 trial participants averaging sixty-four years in age reached basically the
same conclusion. It found that fish, chicken, olive oil, and other
foods rich in omega-3 fatty acids kept participants' memories
sharper than a diet featuring red meat and dairy products. The
one exception was in participants with diabetes: the Mediterranean diet did nothing to slow their memory decline.

The jury is still out on whether the Mediterranean diet can
actually prevent or forestall Alzheimer's. Probably not, is the
short answer. At least, not on its own. The research just says it
may keep your brain a little sharper, and that with early-stage
Alzheimer's patients, it may slow cognitive decline. Why exactly
it has an effect—if it does—is still unclear.

Out there on the Internet, omega-3 fatty acids get all the
credit, but medical researchers are a more cautious bunch. One
theory is that the Mediterranean diet may keep cholesterol levels lower and boost blood vessel health, which in turn may reduce the risk of Alzheimer's and other forms of dementia. Some
say that various benefits of the Mediterranean diet may work
together. "It might be the omegas, the antioxidants, the flavo-
nols, and the large number of vitamins all working together to

have the positive benefit of reducing cognitive impairment," says Kathy McManus, director of the nutrition department at Brigham and Women's Hospital in Boston. "Or it may just be that those who consume a Mediterranean diet tend to be healthier individuals in the first place."

Myself, I don't care that the evidence isn't all in yet. As far as I'm concerned, the scientists can debate the Mediterranean diet for another decade. There's no downside to it—and in particular, no downside to omega-3 fatty acids—and a lot of possible upside for keeping B.'s brain sharper than it would be if we sat around eating steak and potatoes and cheese. That's enough for me.

TIME IS ELASTIC

To a patient with Alzheimer's, five minutes can seem like an hour; an hour can seem like five minutes.

For caregivers, patience is the watchword. I sure learned that! There's no point in correcting or criticizing: a person with Alzheimer's simply can't keep track of time as he or she once did. Putting digital clocks in every room can ease their anxiety. Keeping a large monthly calendar in a common room can be helpful, too: updating it every morning can be a reassuring shared experience.

As I learned how jumbled B.'s sense of time was, I took more care to keep her posted: telling her not just an hour before we were due to be somewhere, but every fifteen minutes.

MILD-STAGE SYMPTOMS

In both the three- and seven-stage models, the start of stage one is so subtle that a patient's family is unlikely to note anything amiss. "No impairment" is the professional term for this first stage. Occasional forgetfulness seems normal—the universal process of aging.

In stage two of the seven-stage model—very mild cognitive decline—a patient may start to forget simple words and familiar names, or to repeat a question over time. Even now, a primary care doctor may not pick up on them, but a loved one may. Those "little signs of difference" start to accumulate. (For a full rundown on both the three- and seven-stage models of Alzheimer's, see pages 146–148.)

Driving

How long to let a person with Alzheimer's drive is an issue both troubling and controversial. The national Alzheimer's Association strikes about the same balance that I did, just by common sense, in the early summer of 2014. I let B. drive but kept a wary eye on her performance. There's no study showing that drivers with mild-stage Alzheimer's have more accidents than others their age. Yet at some point as the disease advances, they clearly must stop driving. The Alzheimer's Association advises caregivers to watch for these warning signs:

- forgetting how to locate familiar places
- failing to observe traffic signs
- making slow or poor decisions in traffic
- driving at an inappropriate speed
- becoming angry or confused while driving

The association also notes that in some states, California among them, doctors must report every Alzheimer's diagnosis to the state health department, which then reports it to the motor vehicles department. Depending on the circumstances, the DMV may revoke the patient's license.

Memory Loss, Repeating Questions

Still unaware that B. had Alzheimer's, I voiced frustration when B. was forgetful and chastised her for asking the same question she'd asked an hour before. In fact, short-term memory loss is one of the first symptoms of Alzheimer's because the part of the brain that governs short-term memory—the hippocampus—is the first to go. Even healthy people lose short-term memories in hours or days: that's all the time a person needs to act on those memories, be they phone numbers or a restaurant address or remembering what clothes one wore the day or two before. With Alzheimer's, those memories just vanish far sooner.

In June 2014, I still had trouble keeping my temper in check. Later, I would learn the caregiver's code for dealing with all shows of memory loss:

Be patient.

Gently repeat what your loved one has forgotten; gently answer the question asked again and again.

Try not to show exasperation; that only deepens your loved one's anxiety and vague awareness that her mind isn't clear.

Find a way to break the feedback loop, by changing the topic of conversation, or perhaps by moving the loved one to another room. If possible, suggest a drive and change the scenery: that works internally as well as externally.

Late to Appointments

The frustration I felt when B. missed meetings was perhaps understandable—if not helpful. As a general note for caregivers, anger and frustration are of no help in dealing with a loved one who has Alzheimer's. They simply provoke hurt and resentment. After a few blown meetings, I learned I had to guide B. to the meetings myself. That didn't make the hurt and resentment go away—those are human reactions that no words of advice can stop a caregiver from feeling.

SLEEPWALKING

It's possible that B.'s episode of sleepwalking was due to dreams that B. thought were real, prompting her actions. Just as likely, she needed to use the bathroom and was disoriented when she awoke in a strange room—enough to wander out into the hotel's corridors in search of it.

Alcohol may have played a role, too. On our trip to New Orleans, B. and I were enjoying festive evenings that included a fair amount of wine. That may have disoriented B. further when she woke up.

I didn't know it then, but cutting back on alcohol is an excellent idea. In fact, cutting out all alcohol, if possible, is a very helpful move. Regular alcohol consumption appears to exacerbate the process by which nerve cells in the brain are killed.

One measure *not* to take with sleepwalking: sleeping pills. Older patients are especially sensitive to sedatives—as are patients with any form of dementia, who may also be on other drugs that interact badly with sedatives. At the least, consult with a doctor first.

Putting a night-light in the bathroom may solve the problem. If a bedroom is on the second floor, a high safety fence across the top of the staircase is a good idea. Daily exercise may fatigue a person enough to help bring on sleep; by the same token, try to prevent daytime napping.

DENIAL

Denial is the flip side of fear, on a coin no one wants to receive. As those coins accumulate, it gets harder to deny the weight of what they mean. Surprisingly, the person with Alzheimer's is sometimes the first to confront the fact of her memory loss. She's still cognizant enough to feel that something's wrong, while her family refuses to see. But that can work in reverse, as the person with Alzheimer's balks at accepting the truth of what's going on. In our case, I guess it was mutual. I started noticing the lapses, but B. didn't deny them.

Either way, dispelling denial is a crucial first step in Alzheimer's care. As Paula Spencer Scott notes in *Surviving Alzheimer's,* deniers often confuse denial with hope: as long as they deny, they reason, there *is* still hope. In fact, as Scott notes, hope and truth can coexist. "Having hope means you're moving forward based on a clear grasp of reality. Denial, in contrast, means avoiding reality because it's too painful to behold."

Those other stages of grief, by the way, are anger, bargaining, depression—and acceptance. All of them are normal reactions to living in Alzheimer's world.

PART 2

THE NEW NORMAL

I don't want to feel like this.

I've always been an emotional person, but it's different now. I cry a lot. I don't know why; I guess sometimes I just feel sad. I feel like I'm misbehaving. I don't want to do that. I want to be nice to my family, but sometimes I can't be. When you're not familiar with what's going on, and everyone around you sees it but you don't, that's hard. People can see how I'm acting more than I can. I don't have the stop-and-gos that I used to have.

So I get mad at Dan. He's the same person I married—I love him, but he's very overbearing. He'll tell me something to do, but then he'll do it himself. We're best friends, and we do have each other's best interests at heart. But Dan is used to taking charge, telling people what to do. And that can be hurtful. I know what's under that. You don't get a lot of respect when you're a black man. You have to fight that much harder. I know what Dan came from—Bedford-Stuyvesant in Brooklyn, where no one gives you a thing—and how he had to scrape to get his first jobs in marketing and sales, and how even later, when people knew who he was, he had to push his way up in industries—TV and radio—where black men were few and far between.

I love my husband, but I like being alone now. Dan will say,

"You have to call your friends." But I've been a social person all my life. When I was a girl I'd cook dinner for my three brothers every night. When I started modeling I was surrounded by people, even more when I opened my first restaurant—and ever since then. I like people—don't get me wrong. But it's sort of a relief not to have to interact with them all. And as much as I love Dan, I need breaks from him, too—especially when it's just the two of us, as it is almost all the time now.

FIVE

New York City

Winter–Spring 2013

B. was too young for Alzheimer's. That's what we thought. Yes, she had grown forgetful. Yes, we had to get her checked out. But whatever was happening, surely it had to relate to a strange physical symptom B. had been feeling for some time. Or so we thought.

B. described it as a sharp, even painful tingling on the left side of her face. It came and went, at first not strongly. Tylenol seemed to help. Perhaps B. had some slightly pinched nerve that would cure itself. Perhaps the problem was stress. Then came the *Today* appearance. Okay, we decided: maybe B. had suffered some kind of mini-stroke. That would account for the tingling on one side of her face, but not the other. Memory loss? That was just a side effect. The stroke's effects would wear off soon enough, and B.'s memory would return.

Looking back, I see what we were doing. Bargaining with fate. A mini-stroke? We could deal with that. Anything but Alzheimer's.

*

Despite that scary moment on the *Today* show, I felt hopeful that B. and I could love, work, and live together for years to come. Whatever her problem was, we'd just solve it and move beyond it.

With that outlook, I landed us a show on SiriusXM satellite radio in early 2013. It was just the two of us interviewing guests for three hours a day, five days a week, about this and that, everything from cooking to politics to the weather. In our first weeks, we got everyone we asked, including Michelle Obama! We had singer Michael Bolton, actor Terrence Howard, former basketball great and ex–New Jersey senator Bill Bradley, and many more. The producers had lists of questions worked up for both of us to ask the guests. When it was B.'s turn, she'd ask the question, and the guest would respond, but then . . . silence. Radio silence. B. just couldn't follow up. I'm a talker, as anyone who knows me will attest. I love to hold forth over a drink as much as the next man, maybe more than most. But even I couldn't handle three hours of interviewing guests while trying to keep B. on track and focusing all my efforts on not having it look like she'd lost the thread. We had a deal with Sirius to earn us six-figure salaries, plus incentives and benchmarks that could bring the pay close to $1 million a year. But without B. there to carry her load, we had to let it go, just weeks after we'd started. It wasn't the only opportunity we'd have to give up. Alzheimer's, as we were learning, changes every expectation you have, and leaves most of them in pieces around you.

Through a friend, we found our way in the spring of 2013 to NYU Langone Medical Center, where a doctor interviewed

B. and concluded that she might be depressed. He prescribed a medical patch, like what a smoker would wear to try to kick the habit, only this one went on B.'s back. The patches felt uncomfortable, left marks, and just made her feel worse.

Next stop was Mount Sinai Hospital. Dr. Jane Martin, an assistant professor of psychiatry at the Mount Sinai School of Medicine, put B. through hours of memory tests. First she asked B. to remember a series of three words, like "red apple ball." Then she asked B. questions like "What's your favorite color?" "What kind of car do you drive?" "What's your birth date?" B. got those just fine, one after another. "Now what was that series of three things I asked you to remember?" the doctor said gently.

B. had no idea.

Her favorite color, her kind of car—those answers were rooted in her long-term memory. The three-word series was short-term memory. B.'s short-term memory was shot.

I could rationalize that easily enough. What sixty-four-year-old could remember a six-word series? Or phone numbers—who can remember ten-digit numbers without a serious effort? But then Dr. Martin put a blank piece of paper in front of B. and asked her to draw the hands of a clock showing 10:45. She couldn't.

That was a shock to me. You don't think of asking your significant other to prove she still knows how to tell time. Still, how had I missed this for so long—months, maybe even a year? Maybe it was partly because B. had a digital watch, and could still read numbers just fine. But also, perhaps, because I had been so self-absorbed and controlling of our work and days that I read the clocks and led the way, and B. just followed along.

Also at Mount Sinai, B. underwent a series of tests for the facial tingling. Doctors put wired electrodes all over her face. I snapped a picture and emailed it to Dana, which probably wasn't a smart idea. It freaked her completely.

The tests, including an MRI, eliminated several possibilities— including stroke. It failed to determine what the tingling was about. Long after the diagnosis, we would still be wondering. Did it trigger the Alzheimer's? Occur as a result? Or was the tingling a totally unrelated issue? To this day our doctors still don't know.

The results of Dr. Martin's cognitive tests left no doubt about our next step. Until recently, the Alzheimer's team at Mount Sinai would have based their diagnosis on these simple cognitive tests, and what we told them: the growing list of small memory lapses, one story after another. For decades that was how doctors had been diagnosing Alzheimer's. That—and one other pretty gruesome test. With a very long and terrifying needle, they would extract a bit of spinal fluid and measure its level of a sticky white protein called amyloid. The less amyloid in the spinal cord, the more there might be in the brain. They knew that amyloid in the brain forms plaques, and that the plaques are associated with dying brain cells—though why amyloid forms those plaques in the first place is the $64,000 question. But amyloid in spinal fluid is still an indirect test, like looking at one of those old fluid-filled glass beakers in your country house kitchen to predict a coming storm.

Now the doctors had a brand-new method to map those plaques in the brain and reach a true, unmistakable diagnosis. They added a radioactive isotope intravenously to B.'s blood that coursed brain-ward through her arteries. For twenty-four hours, we were warned, B. had to stay away from babies and infants—that's how radioactive she was. She couldn't fly: she'd set off the security machines. A Geiger counter set up against her would go berserk. That night she asked me if I wanted to sleep in the spare bedroom. No way, I said. I curled around her as I did every night. Whatever that radioactivity did to B., it could do to me, too.

SIX

NEW YORK CITY

Winter–Spring 2013

The next day, B. went in for what's known as a PET neuro-imaging scan. (*PET* stands for positron emission tomography.) If she had any amyloid plaques, they would show up as clumps of radioactivity. PET imaging for other parts of the body had been around a decade or more, but PET pictures of the brain were brand-new. For neurologists, it was like flicking on a light in a dark room. For the first time, they could see amyloid plaques in a living patient. Until then, the only way to see them was—grim thought—by autopsy.

A day or two later, we went together to see Dr. Martin Goldstein, one of Mount Sinai's dream team of brain doctors. Given his reputation, I expected a large corner office. Instead we found him in a small, dimly lit room crammed with books—a room so small that the four or five chairs sitting there for guests were jammed together. There was so little space between our seats and Dr. Goldstein's desk that my knees bumped up against it.

Dr. Goldstein was in his early forties, though he had the gentle bedside manner of an old-style family doctor. We needed all the comfort he could give. He had studied the PET images of B.'s brain, he said: B. had Alzheimer's. There was no question about it. To us both, it felt like a death sentence. I hadn't known anyone who had Alzheimer's, not personally. My first thought was of President Reagan, so diminished by the end that he couldn't recognize his wife, or remember how he'd served the country. That was a terrifying image.

"Let me show you," Dr. Goldstein said. He turned his computer screen to us so that we could see the brain image on it. There, in soft grays, was B.'s brain. Right in the middle were four or five white irregular shapes, like blobs of Wite-Out. These, Dr. Goldstein explained, were B.'s amyloid plaques. He had his own metaphor for them. "Think of them as potholes in this complex network of roads," he said. "The roads are neurons, going to all parts of the brain. If the roads are clear, the signals on those neurons whiz along to where they're supposed to go. The plaques, unfortunately, are like potholes the signals hit. The potholes throw the signals out of alignment, or maybe off the road altogether."

Medical science, Goldstein added, cannot yet predict what each pothole impact will do to the brain's various functions: speech, short-term memory, executive function, all the different cognitive areas. Nor can it break up the plaques, or keep them from forming. So far, he explained, there's no cure, no reversing the progress of the disease, and no preventive treatment.

Oh, he added—and everybody dies.

"That's the bad news," Dr. Goldstein said.

I stared at him, more angry than shocked. Like . . . there was good news? After that?

"Barbara is at the mildest stage of Alzheimer's," Dr. Goldstein went on. "She has a couple of really good things going for her."

First, B. was still able to function at a relatively high level. She could bathe and dress herself, get around the city, shop for groceries, even cook family dinners. And despite her lapses, there was much she still recalled: long-term memories especially, of her youth, career, and family.

Here was more good news, Dr. Goldstein told us. B. understood she had Alzheimer's. Many people don't. They're not in denial; they just don't think they're sick. As a result, they resist taking drugs that might at least alleviate their symptoms. They don't change their diets or do regular exercise. Worst of all, they can't talk about their illness with their loved ones. Often they get angry, not knowing that their anger, too, is part of the disease.

That day, Dr. Goldstein laid out what the daily intake of pills would be. There are, he explained, two kinds of drugs to date developed for Alzheimer's. One works to slow the breakdown of a chemical in the brain related to memory and learning. That chemical is called acetylcholine, so the drugs that try to protect it are called acetylcholinesterase inhibitors (or AChEIs for short). Of the three in that class that are on the market, the one Dr. Goldstein prescribed for B. was Aricept. The other kind of drug focuses on another brain chemical, glutamate, also important for memory and learning. There's only one drug of that kind, so that was the one B. got. It's called Namenda.

We shouldn't get our hopes up, Dr. Goldstein told us. At best, these drugs might diminish B.'s symptoms a little: her memory loss, her language issues, her cognitive decline. Not much, though, and not for long. When we got home, I looked them up. Here's what Namenda's manufacturer says on its website: "There is no evidence that Namenda or an AChEI prevents or slows the underlying disease process in patients with Alzheimer's disease."

Great!

No one had to tell us that Alzheimer's often brings on depression: B.'s moods were all too familiar by now, just identified, rather than mysterious. For that Dr. Goldstein prescribed Wellbutrin, a powerful antidepressant that might improve her moods—but also might lead to seizures. (To counteract that danger, Dr. Goldstein prescribed an antiseizure drug called Topamax.) For general health, Dr. Goldstein added the multivitamin Coenzyme Q10 (CoQ10) and B vitamins. Plus aspirin for stroke prevention.

Nowhere on that list was an anti-Alzheimer's drug. No "take this and keep it from getting worse." The doctors didn't have a drug like that—not yet. Nor did they have a cure, or a vaccine to prevent it altogether. The word Dr. Goldstein kept using was *managed*. Experts in the field are hopeful that Alzheimer's may become a managed disease, so that a combination of drugs, vitamins, diet, and exercise may keep a mild-stage patient's condition from progressing.

Sticking to a Mediterranean diet and getting regular exercise were just as important as the drugs, we were told, to keeping Alzheimer's at bay. With any luck, they would help keep

B. stable—long enough for the breakthrough drug to come along.

Mount Sinai Hospital is on upper Fifth Avenue, north of the fancy buildings but still overlooking the upper part of Central Park. When we left Dr. Goldstein's office, we walked down the park side of the avenue awhile, not saying much. B. held my arm with two hands, as if a storm might sweep her away. I felt awful for her, and overwhelmed, the word *Alzheimer's* just flashing in my mind like a big red neon sign.

But to my surprise, I also felt a wave of relief. Knowing was better than not knowing. A diagnosis let us focus. Now, at least, we could do whatever there was to do. Dr. Goldstein had mentioned new drug trials; we could enroll B. in those. A new diet—hell, yes. If anyone could embrace a new diet, it was B. Food was what she *did*. As for exercise, that was easy. B. had always been relatively fit. We'd get really fit now.

Maybe I was selfish to think this, but part of my relief was in knowing that all those angry moments we'd had over the last two years weren't signs our marriage was falling apart. That wasn't B. talking, all those times.

It was the disease.

SEVEN

New York City

Spring 2013

In our twenty-one-year marriage, I had acted not just as B.'s husband and best friend but as her business partner. I did the negotiating, got the book contracts and magazine deals and product endorsements. Now I had a new role: caregiver.

I knew that hiring someone to help would make the most sense. I just didn't want to do it. I couldn't imagine a stranger in our Manhattan apartment, let alone our Sag Harbor house. I also felt no one could care better for B. than me. Which was true. But I hadn't anticipated how all-consuming that new job would be as the months wore on. All you caregivers out there— you know what I mean. It's *hard*.

For starters, I now did most of the house stuff: shopping and cooking, keeping the kitchen clean, and picking up after B. If I had meetings outside the apartment, I had to be sure B. would remember to eat while I was gone. Usually she didn't.

A regular stop on my rounds was the B. Smith's restaurant on Theatre Row. The restaurant was sputtering but still going, in part because B. could still stop by and talk up the tables. Unfortunately, the B. Smith's restaurant in Washington, D.C., had closed earlier in 2013. Despite the good business we were doing, the rent was just too high for a location in Union Station, elegant as the station's restoration might be. As for our Sag Harbor site, it would last the summer of 2013, but I saw no way to justify keeping it through the next winter, a season when all Hamptons businesses struggle to stay alive. There, too, a high rent crimped our profits, and our biggest draw—B. herself—no longer felt able to talk up the summer crowd night after night.

In all three restaurants, B. had been my full-time partner. She was at best a part-time partner now, and in a very limited way. It was like having one hand tied behind my back. Thank God we had all those B. Smith products in Bed Bath & Beyond and a strong relationship with the company.

One of my largest frustrations had nothing to do with the business. B. was losing her intellectual curiosity. She couldn't get through a book. Movies and plays and the rest of the arts were simply a blur to her now. That was hard for me. I like a woman who's engaged with the world, who has opinions. If they're different from my opinions, all the better. A sharp debate creates tension, and tension creates sexual desire. When B. and I started dating, we could spend the whole evening debating the war with Iraq—the *first* President Bush's war—and let me tell you, the end of an evening like that was hot. I had to accept that that whole dynamic was pretty much gone, and not coming back.

Which is not to say that sex was gone from our marriage. It was just at a very different vibe.

At sixty-four, B. was still a beautiful woman—a world-class stunner, with that fabulous smile, perfect complexion, and gorgeous figure. You look at the picture on this book and tell me: Does she not look at least fifteen years younger than her age? The desire I felt for her when we met was all-consuming; I still felt desire for her now, but on B.'s side the passion was gone. She loved me, but in a distracted way. She cuddled, but that was about it. The lover I knew was gone, replaced by a new, more muted version of the woman I had married.

To be totally up front about it, I had my own issues. I was a veteran of prostate cancer. To the outside world, B. and I were as glamorous a couple as you could find. Privately we were struggling well before B.'s first memory lapse—before I even heard the word *caregiver,* much less knew what it involved. I got through the prostate surgery—the *right* way, which I won't elaborate on here; that's for another book—and I recovered, so as that scare eased, I was up for a little flirting from my wife, the kind that used to be as natural as breathing. We were still breathing, but flirting was just one of the many things we'd lost with Alzheimer's.

Instead, I had to do all the initiating. B. was sweet and gentle—affectionate, too. Just not responsive. Quiet—I guess that's the word that puts it best. Most of the time I resented the disease, but not always. Sometimes I resented B., too.

Now that we had the diagnosis, I tried viewing the physical side of our marriage in a new way. As a person with Alzheimer's, B. lived more and more in the present. My challenge, as her husband and caregiver, was to immerse myself in the present tense with her. Not to expect her to remember what we'd planned for the day, or what we did the day before. Just to be there with her. And what in our day-to-day lives is more present tense than sex? In those moments of connection, all else is forgotten and falls away. How different, then, is making love when one of those two people has Alzheimer's? Before and after— yes. Very different. But not in the act itself.

B. couldn't join me in my world of past and future tense. But I could join her in *her* world, and make her happy there—and in so doing, make myself happy, too.

The doctors and therapists who work with Alzheimer's care- givers have a phrase for this. *Joining the journey.* Your loved one with Alzheimer's is on a journey you cannot block or prevent. You can't even pull her aside for a while, trying to shake her into remembering what seems so obvious to you. All you can do is join the journey—to share with her each next moment of being, even as each next moment displaces the last. Making love, I've come to realize, is the ultimate in-the-moment experience for a couple coping with Alzheimer's.

So is our time together after making love. That's the one time left when we still converse with real intimacy. It's when B.'s in- nermost feelings come out. It's when she'll say, "I know you love me, and I know you care, and I know I'm lucky to have you."

I feel that same depth of intimacy for her, even knowing the person beside me isn't quite the person she was. She's still B. to me—still beautiful, with all that same physical topography I know so well, and the same taste of her lips, and same sweet smell of her I've known so long I can't imagine not knowing it anymore.

EIGHT

New York City

Spring 2013

Not long after we got B.'s diagnosis, we went back to Mount Sinai to meet Dr. Sam Gandy, the hospital's top dog in Alzheimer's research—a neurologist *and* a psychiatrist. He was the guy who, along with Dr. Martin Goldstein, would be following B.'s case.

I'll say this about Alzheimer's: it sure is a bonding experience. Start telling people Alzheimer's has hit your family, and damned if almost everyone you meet doesn't have a story of how it hit theirs. Dr. Gandy was no exception. He told us about growing up in rural South Carolina with a grandmother whose Alzheimer's grew quite extreme by the time Sam was ten years old. Sam's grandmother didn't get forgetful or withdrawn. Instead, she got hostile and agitated, and just took off down the road, to be picked up, sooner or later, by the police—and then reclaimed by the family at the police station.

Sam's grandmother was institutionalized sooner than she would have been today. Families didn't try to keep their addled

grandparents at home if their behavior became difficult to control, or if, as often happened, they became incontinent. Sam's
grandmother was increasingly psychotic, which is a not-unusual
symptom of Alzheimer's in its later stages. Eventually her family had to put her in the state-run Hall Psychiatric Institute, in
Columbia, South Carolina. Sam and his parents would visit her
weekly. She wouldn't recognize them. She knew she had family;
she just didn't know who they were.

As a kid of ten or eleven, Dr. Gandy told us, he would get
fidgety on these visits, and so would wander off around the hospital to see what he could see. Virtually everyone in that hospital
had late-stage Alzheimer's. Some were tied to their wheelchairs,
others tied to their beds. Almost all had vacant stares, or were
babbling to themselves. The hospital staff got to know Sam, and
the doctors would explain each patient's condition to him.

In most other ways, Sam's grandmother was healthy as a
horse. She lived fifteen years with Alzheimer's, and Sam kept
visiting, right up through medical school. He didn't know at
first that he wanted to be a neurologist and study the disease
that took his grandmother. For a while he just knew he loved
research. But he found himself fascinated by the mystery of why
and how the brain began to destroy itself. He went on to earn
both an MD and PhD, and to devote his life to unlocking that
mystery.

"I still find it thrilling, all the more so now that we're getting
so close—not to a cure, but to stopping this dreadful disease
from progressing," Dr. Gandy told us. "I think there's a more
than even chance we'll get there by 2020, and I think it's entirely feasible that B. will still be a mild-stage patient, with a
decent quality of life, when we do."

Dr. Gandy told us there was new excitement about the success of vitamin E in slowing the progress of Alzheimer's, especially in mild-to-moderate-stage patients. "It's not great, but it's real," he told us. "That's what progress usually looks like with a tough disease like Alzheimer's: small steps that add up. Until now we had lots of conflicting research about Vitamin E. No longer." Now a consensus had formed: Vitamin E did seem to help.

Another small but significant step was the development of new drugs to stimulate the formation of nerve cells in the brain. The drugs didn't prevent amyloid plaques, or the protein "tangles," called tau, that actually seem to kill cells. "But they help restore or maintain function in the face of the disease," Dr. Gandy told us. Not a treatment, not a cure, just a bit of help for the brain—I was getting the picture.

There *were* new drug trials, and B. would qualify for one or more of those, Dr. Gandy assured us. The one he had in mind was for an insulin-based drug called T-817MA. There was evidence that people with type 2 diabetes and a resistance to processing insulin were at high risk for developing Alzheimer's. A particular gene seemed to cause both insulin resistance *and* Alzheimer's. "So there's been a small trial for patients who have some related symptoms, with insulin given intranasally," Dr. Gandy explained. "It improves their memory by getting insulin to the brain." Again, it wasn't a cure, or even a treatment. And for B., who had neither diabetes nor high blood sugar, it was a bit of a stretch. But it might help. All B. had to do in order to qualify was take Aricept for three months. It would alleviate a little of the fog of Alzheimer's, enough that the researchers could more accurately measure the effect of the new insulin drug on her.

Dr. Gandy cautioned us that one new drug was almost certainly not the answer to Alzheimer's. Other drugs were needed. Unfortunately, the funding for Alzheimer's research was shockingly minimal. Heart disease, cancer, and AIDS got billions of research dollars each year from the National Institutes of Health, and more from national nonprofits like the American Cancer Society. The NIH's annual budget for Alzheimer's was, by comparison, minuscule: $400 million. There were plenty of good ideas to try, he said. The problem was resources. "People spend years raising the money, then five years to get the trial done. A decade here, a decade there, pretty soon your life's over!"

Meanwhile, the problem continued to grow. "Almost half of Americans over eighty-five years old have Alzheimer's," Dr. Gandy said, his frustration all too clear. "The disease will cost every one of those patients an average of one million dollars: about fifty to one hundred thousand dollars a year for home care, not to mention drugs, over the ten-year average that a patient lives with the disease." Multiply that by 5.2 million people with Alzheimer's and what do you get? A trillion dollars and change. "We have this expensive common problem," Dr. Gandy said soberly. "It's been there for a while and we weren't paying attention to it. Now the aging of the baby boomers means the numbers keep going up."

It was like some secret club we hadn't even known existed. And now we, too, were members. The dues? Up to a hundred thousand dollars a year. Length of membership? Eight to ten years on average. The emotional cost of it all to us as a family?

Priceless.

LESSONS LEARNED

Basic Personality Changes

Early-onset Alzheimer's patients tend to fall into one of four common personality types. I was relieved to know that B. in her mild stage, at the start of summer 2013, was a perfect example of the best of the bunch. She was—and still is—good-natured and open to suggestion most of the time. She knows she has Alzheimer's, and sometimes gets depressed about it, but more often than not her spirits are up. That is a blessing.

The other three personality types are far more challenging:

Apathetic

As a mild-stage patient begins to struggle with tasks or thoughts or sentences that are in some way complex, so grows the inclination to abandon the effort. The patient is losing the part of his brain that governs what's called executive function. Antidepressant medicine may help; physical exercise is certainly helpful, as are small household tasks that the loved one can feel some pride in mastering, like organizing kitchen cabinets or vacuuming. I do see some apathy in B., but having a task, or a plan of any kind, tends to bring her spirits back up.

Depressed

Often the awareness of one's worsening condition, and the helplessness one feels to affect it, can increase tensions and antisocial behavior, which in turn feed depression and anxiety.

I see that in B. maybe more now than I used to, but so far exercise and satisfying tasks like cooking help.

Paranoid and Frightened

As Alzheimer's loosens a patient's perceptions and sense of reality, she may create new realities to fill what's missing. A handyman who's come to fix the stove may suddenly seem an intruder; a spouse may seem a stranger. Thankfully, B. hasn't had any interludes like that.

These personality changes are hard to accept—believe me, I know—but as a caregiver you learn to react with gentleness, to sympathize but not to correct, and, when possible, to take the loved one to a new environment—an ice-cream parlor, say—to dispel the paranoia.

THE POWER OF LOVE

In a San Diego suburb in the early 1980s, a pioneer in Alzheimer's research, George Glenner, together with his wife, Joy, started the country's first private home-care facility for Alzheimer's patients. The Glenners were doing cutting-edge lab research to understand what the disease was, and what caused it, in the hope of finding a cure. But they saw the need for immediate, hands-on help for Alzheimer's patients, and turned a Hillcrest cottage into the Alzheimer's Family Center. As the Glenners began tending their first guests, they let instinct guide them. The best thing they could do, they saw, was to alleviate their patients' stress, however they could: to be soothing, supportive—and loving. Joy Glenner came to believe that a treatment for Alzheimer's lay right at hand. "It's a glue called love. You can have a very disoriented or combative person, and love can help calm them."

THE DAILY INTAKE OF PILLS

There are no drugs that cure a patient of Alzheimer's; there are not even any drugs that keep it in check. All we have are four drugs that help treat Alzheimer's symptoms.

Three of those drugs take the same approach, boosting the brain's supply of acetylcholine, a neurotransmitter that communicates signals from neuron to neuron. Alzheimer's damages those neurotransmitters. With more acetylcholine coursing through their brains, many patients find they can think more clearly and maintain better memories. B. was prescribed the one called Aricept (donepezil). Others are Razadyne (galantamine) and Exelon (rivastigmine). All work best in patients with early-stage Alzheimer's.

A fourth drug, Namenda (memantine), regulates the action of another neurotransmitter called glutamate, which is central to learning and memory. In another context glutamate is a common food ingredient, conferring flavor, and helps the process of metabolism; in moderate amounts, it's essential to health. In the brain, glutamate plays a key role. It attaches to cell surface "docking sites" called NMDA receptors, allowing for the transmission of calcium, which enables learning and spurs memory. Alzheimer's gums up the process, leading to excess glutamate and calcium, which can damage the cells. Namenda helps control this runaway process by partially blocking the NMDA receptors so that not too much calcium goes from cell to cell. The good news is that the U.S. Food and Drug Administration has allowed it to be prescribed for patients with moderate to severe Alzheimer's. The bad news is that it works for just a few months, if at all.

With all four drugs, only about half the patients who take them see improvement. And as they say in all those drug commercials on TV, some patients experience serious side effects.

ALTERNATIVE MEDICATIONS

For some years, natural substances thought to enhance memory have offered hope for Alzheimer's patients. One that we've tried is ginkgo biloba, derived from the leaves of the plant. Ginkgo has been used for centuries in Chinese traditional medicine as an antioxidant and anti-inflammatory agent, and is thought to keep brain cells healthy and functioning. Early clinical studies showed mild improvement in cognitive function for older patients with Alzheimer's and other kinds of dementia. Unfortunately, a recent large-scale trial conducted by branches of the National Institutes of Health has disappointed all of us who thought it might be a magic bullet. Some three thousand participants aged seventy-five or older, some with no signs of dementia, others with mild impairment, took either ginkgo extract or a placebo regularly for six years. The bottom line: just as many members in the ginkgo group got Alzheimer's over those six years as in the placebo group.

I'm sorry to say that it's more of the same with a moss extract called huperzine A, another ancient Chinese medicine. Huperzine A appeared to have the same effect as those three drugs that boosted acetylcholine. Unfortunately, in its first large-scale US trial, run by the Alzheimer's Disease Cooperative

Study (ADCS), it performed no better than a placebo in slowing the progress of the disease in mild to moderate cases. The Alzheimer's Association now actually warns against its usage. Available over the counter as a dietary supplement, it may have harmful side effects, especially if taken in addition to FDA-approved Alzheimer's drugs.

The word on omega-3 fatty acids, mentioned earlier, is more promising. Omega-3s, a kind of polyunsaturated fatty acid, are thought to help prevent heart disease and stroke, and are included in various over-the-counter food supplements. Some studies have shown that omega-3s can help counteract Alzheimer's and other forms of dementia: healthy brain cells contain the omega-3 called DHA, and omega-3 supplements may boost their ability to fight the inflammation associated with Alzheimer's. (As amyloid forms plaques, it causes inflammation, and that, as Rudy Tanzi notes in his Foreword, becomes a vicious circle: more amyloid, more inflammation, more amyloid. Inflammation is also associated with the tau tangles found in brain cells under siege.) Again, large-scale clinical trials have tempered expectations. One found that DHA offered no more help to individuals with mild to moderate Alzheimer's than a placebo. But a second trial using only healthy older adults showed that those who took DHA scored better on memory tests over time than those given placebos.

So maybe it's a matter of taking the omega-3s earlier—like maybe years earlier, as a preventive measure. Or perhaps the omega-3s found in foods work in tandem with antioxidants or other substances to sharpen memory. No study has yet proved exactly how omega-3s work in the body, and whether they actively work against Alzheimer's, as either a treatment or preventive measure. All I know is that unlike huperzine A, omega-3s appear to have no downside. Until that downside is found, B. and I will stick by our omega-3–rich Mediterranean diet and hope for the best.

THE PROBLEM WITH ALTERNATIVES

All drugs are subjected to three phases of federally monitored tests. In Phase I, a drug is given to a small group of patients. If results are promising *and* if the drug is deemed safe—then it's on to the larger Phase II, and finally Phase III, usually with thousands of trial participants. The larger the group, of course, the more likely that some dangerous side effect may appear. All it takes is a bad side effect in one or two of those thousands of participants to imperil a new drug's chances. When it comes to alternative or natural medicines for Alzheimer's, most fall short when put through three-phase trials. Most, for that matter, turn out to have no efficacy at all.

Often, when makers of those alternatives get bad news from clinical trials, they bail out of the process and call their products "supplements," not drugs. In natural supplements stores, for example, you can buy a "medical food" called Axona. Its chief ingredient is caprylic acid, which in the body breaks down into substances that may act like a glucose supplement, strengthening brain cell capacity after Alzheimer's has reduced natural glucose levels. A Phase II study with a limited number of volunteers appeared to show that Axona at least worked better than a placebo. But according to the Alzheimer's Association, the manufacturer of Axona has declined to conduct large-scale Phase III studies. Instead, by claiming that it is merely a supplement, it has been able to market Axona without performing those tests. The Alzheimer's Association has, as a result, expressed concern about Axona. Coconut oil, another source of caprylic acid, has had anecdotal success, but it has not been put to any formal tests.

Another kind of "medical food," called VIVImind, uses an amino acid called tramiprosate, found in seaweed. Unlike Axona, VIVImind was subjected to Phase III trials as a possible Alzheimer's drug treatment. When results proved inconclusive, the manufacturer withdrew it and chose instead to market VIVImind as a "medical food" like Axona. Neither the FDA nor the Alzheimer's Association has recommended its use.

Coenzyme Q10 is an antioxidant that B. and I take every day, because it, like Axona, has had anecdotal success in slowing the progression of Alzheimer's. It's a natural substance in the body, essential for normal cell reactions; synthesized and sold as a natural supplement, CoQ10, or ubiquinone, has been tested for Alzheimer's and found to have no discernible benefit. The Alzheimer's Association warns that in excess amounts, it could have harmful effects, but B. and I just take the recommended dosage, and hope that it does have some healthful effects on our energy and memory.

Coral calcium is another over-the-counter supplement that needs no FDA approval because it's not marketed as a drug. Its manufacturers claim that it's derived from the shells of dead coral reef organisms, and that its calcium has various health benefits, among them promoting the production of calcium in the brain, which in turn staves off Alzheimer's. The Federal Trade Commission has filed a formal complaint against the makers and distributors of coral calcium, noting that there's no proof it has any benefits at all.

Phosphatidylserine is a lipid that surrounds nerve cells. The theory here is that phosphatidylserine extracted from various sources may keep those cells from breaking down. Supplements based on lipids from soy extracts have not been tested, and the FDA declares that no evidence of their efficacy yet exists. The Alzheimer's Association recommends not using it.

Doctors tend to feel the same. Along with one of the four symptom-treating drugs, a doctor will usually prescribe simple vitamins and, depending on the patient's frame of mind, perhaps an antidepressant, as ours did for B.—but not any of those alternative approaches.

Lest all this sound even more discouraging than it is, let me end this section of alternative therapies on a high note: BDNF, or, if you want the whole tongue-twister, brain-derived neuro-trophic factor. It's not a supplement sold over the counter but a protein found in our brains. More BDNF in the brain appears to mean better brain health—better enough to reduce Alzheimer's in 50 percent of a group of older adults followed for ten years in a study by researchers from Boston University. But I'll let the doctor who's doing the most to get BDNF to market explain his hopes for it in a later chapter.

PREVENTING BURNOUT

At the top of the list of specific tips for caregivers is *not to burn out,* since that of course helps neither party. How to do it? Don't forget to give care to yourself.

- Get enough rest.
- Take enough time off to recharge.
- Get family members and friends to help.

- When the need arises for a home health-care worker, don't ignore it.

OTHER IDEAS THAT HAVE HELPED US

- Read the literature; learn as much as you can about the disease; get in touch with your local branch of the Alzheimer's Association.
- In conversational groups of three or more, don't treat your loved one as if she doesn't exist, and don't refer to her in the third person.
- Don't try to finish a loved one's sentences. Give her time to respond. If she can't retrieve her thought after a long pause, gently prompt her with what you think she's trying to say.
- Avoid being condescending or critical, at all costs. It's debilitating, and simply doesn't work. Try to ask questions that can be answered with a yes or no. Instead of "What shall we wear today?" try "How about these black pants?"

Above all, never lose sight of the dignity within the human being who has the disease.

SEX AND SEXUAL BEHAVIORS

Nothing is the same with Alzheimer's—including sex. So far, we have managed to maintain a semblance of the sexual relations we shared before our lives changed. Not all couples are so lucky. A wife may slip into the covers beside her husband and ask why he's there in bed with her: a buzzkill for even an ardent partner. She may, instead, engage in sex with her husband, only to lose all memory, a few minutes later, of having done so:

another dampener, for sure. B. has not acted in those ways—not yet—though I've certainly learned that sex with Alzheimer's means more cuddling and touching than intercourse.

As the disease progresses, a patient's interest in sex will likely diminish, increasing a partner's stress and frustration as a caregiver. Unfortunately, there's no easy answer for that. Other patients may show a heightened interest in sex, creating problems of a different kind. In *Living with Alzheimer's,* from the Chicken Soup for the Soul series, a support group counselor recalls a new member raising her hand to say she had an odd issue to report. "The problem is that we will have sex in the morning and by lunchtime he forgets that we had sex. He will approach me longingly and say, 'Honey, c'mon, we haven't had sex for days. He's insatiable.' " There was, as the counselor recalls, a moment of grave silence before someone else cried, "I wish I had that problem!" and the whole group collapsed in laughter.

Occasionally, a patient will exhibit inappropriate behavior, such as touching himself or herself, even masturbating. Alarming and embarrassing as this behavior may be, family and friends need to recognize that the patient hasn't lost his sense of decorum or become some sort of sex maniac. This is the disease in action, not the patient. I'm relieved to say that hasn't been our issue, but what the experts say to do makes complete sense to me. Gently advise the patient that that's not what we do, and quickly suggest a more constructive activity! Preparing a meal together, perhaps, or taking a walk.

PART 3

PUTTING ASIDE
PRIDE AND PRIVACY

I'll tell you the biggest problem for me: trying to remember things Dan or Dana tells me. In the beginning, I felt like there were things happening, and I needed to write them down to remember them, and so I did. I have a little book for that. Dan can tell me something and I might not remember it ten minutes later. But I try to by writing it down in that book. I'll even write it on my hand, if I don't have the book right there.

Usually I keep the book in my handbag. But then I have to remember where my handbag is. I started misplacing it, so now I have it down to a good science. I just carry it with me wherever I go, from room to room. My mother taught me that a lady always carries a handbag, and so I do. I still do.

I try to have a routine. When we're in Manhattan, I take Bishop out for walks every day to Central Park. Most evenings, I walk to the restaurant, from our apartment on Fifty-Ninth street down to Forty-Sixth Street: it's on Theatre Row, between Eighth and Ninth avenues. Until last fall I was involved with all aspects of the business, including talking to every single customer who came in each night. I loved doing that, and I did it no matter how I felt— whether I had a cold or flu, no sleep the night before, whatever. I know this sounds like boasting, but the waiters loved having me *there even more than the customers: the tips were always larger. I don't do that as often, but I try. I still know how important that is.*

That's in the city. On weekends in Sag Harbor, I'll take Bishop for long walks on the beach. I feel like I know where I'm going on my walks, and I have no trouble getting back. You can't get lost on a beach, right? But I'm conscious that I'm telling myself, "Okay, here's where we're going, and here's how we're going home." That helps. If I don't do that, it's more likely that I'll get depressed. Because who wants to forget what you're supposed to remember?

NINE

NEW YORK CITY/
SAG HARBOR

Summer–Fall 2013

With the diagnosis we were, at least, through the WTF period. We knew what B. had, and we had drugs to deal with it. Well—not deal with it, but make it more tolerable. Only B. kept losing the drugs. "Did you take your medicine?" I would demand.

B. would hang her head. "No," she would say in a small voice, "I can't find it."

About the sixth time that happened I blew up. "This is bullshit," I said. It wasn't the first time I lost my temper with B., and it wouldn't be the last. I knew that B. couldn't help losing the drugs. I knew I should be patient when she did. Holding a person with Alzheimer's to the same standards of responsibility and remembering as everyone else is absurd, but it happens when the person in question is your spouse. One of the hardest lessons to learn about Alzheimer's is that your loved one is only partly the person she once was. The disease is taking over, directing her behavior. When she does something that seems disrespectful, or sloppy, or when she lashes out, or simmers in silence, that's not your loved one. That's the disease.

Of course, you find yourself having the same expectations of her that you did before, and so you react accordingly. *That's* the bullshit. I'm sure some caregivers can put aside those expectations right away. I'm sorry to say I wasn't one of them. I vented at B., and then felt awful about it. In retrospect, I wish I'd reached out sooner for help. Instead I thought I could do it all myself. That, I've since learned, is an all-too-common syndrome for caregivers. Going it alone doesn't make you a hero. It just wears you down, and burns you out, so that you can't be the caregiver you need to be.

We had days when the drugs were misplaced; we had others when the drugs B. took seemed to make her hallucinate. One in particular—Wellbutrin, for depression—got her thinking there were shadowy figures in the corner. Wellbutrin agitated her, too—made her hostile and restless. Once she saw her mother and started talking to her, convinced that her mother was standing right in front of her. I'm not saying it was the drug's fault, exactly: more than once, B. got hold of a vial of the stuff, forgot she'd taken a pill earlier that day, and took another, or maybe three. Finally, I snatched the responsibility of the drugs from her, put them in a safe, secret place, and dispensed them to her one by one. At least she was getting the right drugs at the proper dosage. But now, in addition to being her pharmacist, I was shopping for groceries, cooking every meal, cleaning up after, doing the laundry, not to mention being B.'s clothes consultant every time she got dressed. And all this on top of my day job! It isn't easy asking for help when you're a strong, black man from Bedford-Stuyvesant, brought up to fend for yourself. But ultimately, with Alzheimer's, you have no choice.

Dana, our daughter, was the one who came to our rescue. In October 2013, she moved up from Washington, D.C., to live with us in Manhattan. She was twenty-seven, fully independent, years past living at home. She even had a boyfriend. But she could hear my frustration, and she knew how often B. was repeating herself. I don't remember if I asked, or she volunteered. Her parents just needed her, and that was that. Together we were learning a hard lesson about Alzheimer's: that it changes everyone's plans. One person has the disease, but everyone in the family is affected. No one's life is ever the same.

With Dana came her huge Italian mastiff, Bishop—so called because he's mostly black with a white cross on his chest. If I had rolled my eyes at the thought of such a large dog for Dana in D.C., I rolled them no more. Bishop was a godsend. Overnight he became B.'s guard dog. Somehow he just sensed her vulnerability. He watched her every move, radiated love and devotion, and curled up beside her. For B., walking Bishop in Central Park became the high point of her day. If someone recognized her and came up to say hello, Bishop blocked her protectively. I felt sorry for any mugger who might think he had a vulnerable target in B. That mugger had another thing coming.

It was, like Rick says to the police chief at the end of *Casablanca,* the start of a beautiful friendship. B. loves Bishop as much as he loves her, and she's his caregiver, too—so much so that after a month or so back in New York, Dana officially gave Bishop to B. Nothing could have made B. happier. And when you think about it, what could be better for a person with Alzheimer's than a loving service dog? Not only do they share the joy of unconditional love: they're partners in the present tense. Bishop is oblivious to B.'s memory lapses; and all that matters to her is that he's there for her in the moment, always loving, never judging. The only problem with this beautiful friendship, I came to see, is that B. as Bishop's self-appointed caregiver often forgets when she's last fed him, and how much. Sometimes he gets two meals a day, sometimes four. We took to putting a can of sardines in with his chow: good for dogs as well as humans. So now he may get one can of sardines a day . . . or four. To my knowledge, he's never complained.

Dana hadn't imagined that at twenty-seven, she would be telling her parents what to do. By the time she moved back in, though, we were so frazzled that we needed her to do just that. She took control of the drugs: from then on, she hid them from both of us, and doled them out to B. as needed. I stopped blaming B. for losing them, and B. stopped getting upset when she did. Dana started doing a lot of the cooking, too: big one-pot meals with leftovers for the next day. Dana had grown up watching B. cook mouthwatering southern food, and had come to be a good cook herself. B. was still cooking, too, but sometimes she overseasoned her dishes, forgetting she'd seasoned them already. Sometimes, too, if I had meetings away from the apartment, B. might forget to eat. Now Dana was there to be sure she did.

Most important, Dana took over the B. Smith's restaurant on West Forty-Sixth Street. Managing the restaurant was well beyond B. now; she struggled just to greet the guests a few nights a week and keep the place aglow. The first night Dana went down with her to see how she could help, she saw that a little part of B. was lost—a part Dana had thought she still had. Still, Dana tried to stay upbeat about it. At least B. still came to the restaurant: it was still B. Smith's. And in so many essential ways, B. was still the parent she'd always been to Dana.

Like all families, ours had its own complicated dynamic. B. is Dana's stepmother. Dana was five when B. entered her life, and what a happy miracle that was for Dana and me both. Her birth mother and I had divorced after a very volatile marriage, and Dana hadn't seen much of Jocelyn after that, not on any regular basis. B. was the one who came to the games: field hockey and basketball, soccer and lacrosse; Dana was quite the jock. From her birth mother, Dana had inherited a slightly manic spirit, and her relationship with Jocelyn was contentious. B. was the great equalizer, as Dana put it: cool, calm, and collected, always gentle and solicitous.

The way Dana saw it, B. had managed her life, and now Dana was returning the favor. When someone in your family gets Alzheimer's, we were learning, you have to start to think not just about managing them but about managing your own life in tandem with theirs: building in the time to be a daily caregiver, but also scheduling time off to replenish yourself and be able to help your loved one the next day.

One night we were talking about that after B. had gone to bed. I wasn't good at the downtime part yet—taking time for myself, "managing" it into the schedule. Dana agreed. "You suck at it, Dad," she told me. One thing about Dana: you get the truth every time. "But I'm not so great at it, either," she added. "In all those books about Alzheimer's they talk about 'managing,' like it's managing a checkbook." She shook her head. "I've come to hate that word *managing*."

B. had outbursts now. That was entirely new. I was the one she blew up at. Invariably, Dana took her side. "Why are you egging her on?" she would exclaim. I wasn't doing anything, I would protest, like a kid whose mother was on his case. I was just telling B. where her handbag was, or asking if she'd eaten anything yet that day.

"It's not what you say, it's how you say it," Dana would say. "If I wasn't your daughter, I might punch you."

She was right. I kept trying to be patient and understanding, but irritation crept into my tone.

Just as out of character for B. were the mild profanities she sometimes used now. One day I had a friend take B. to her hairdresser in Sag Harbor. Historically in black communities, hairdressers worked out of their homes; there weren't any storefront salons for women in the South—or North, for that matter, except in Harlem. Decades later, Sag Harbor's black women still go to the hairdresser's house, affluent as their families might be. They like the custom. Also, as in the Deep South, the hairdresser's is where gossip flows.

B. didn't know the women under the other hair dryers that day, but they knew her, and they noticed that this household name known for her sweetness and light was swearing like a sailor. Later, the girlfriend who had brought her to the hairdresser's took her to lunch at a restaurant in Bridgehampton. B. was happy, animated—and using language that the friend had never heard her use before. Before Alzheimer's, I was the one who did the cursing for the whole family. I'd never heard B. curse.

That's a funny thing about Alzheimer's, I was starting to realize: it makes you act in ways you never did before—both the person with it and the family living it. Every day is like the beginning of a new normal.

Here was another new aspect of B.: she started raiding the kitchen late at night for sugary snacks. She'd never done that before. Nor was she ever less than neat. Now I'd pad into the kitchen in the morning and see crumbs on the counter, an opened package of cereal, or an empty pint of ice cream. I told her how bad the sugar is for her: not just for all the obvious reasons, but for Alzheimer's, too. She told me she was sorry and said it wouldn't happen again, but I could tell she was just saying that. She didn't even remember having the snack.

TEN

NEW YORK CITY

Winter–Spring 2014

One day about five months after the diagnosis, we went to Mount Sinai for a checkup with Dr. Goldstein. Once again we filed into his tiny, dimly lit office, took two of the scrunched-together chairs, and struggled for legroom against his desk. Once again he turned his computer screen toward us so that we could see B.'s brain scan with its amyloid plaques.

"Last time we tried Wellbutrin/bupropion XL, two hundred milligrams for executive cognition," Dr. Goldstein began, addressing his remarks to B. "The cognitive symptoms were taking a toll on your morale. That was leading to depression symptoms."

B. nodded.

"Separate from the depression, Alzheimer's can produce distraction . . . keep you from focusing. That can make your memory worse. Also, depression becomes a risk factor in the progression of Alzheimer's." He paused. "Looking back in terms of your spirits overall, how do things seem? Better? Worse?"

"Better," B. whispered. She started tearing up.

"Some tearfulness is to be expected," Dr. Goldstein said. "If things make you sad, you should feel sad, but I want you to be in control of those experiences." Had B. felt in control of her feelings? he asked.

"Sometimes," B. said. "In general. I feel good, but I'm a little emotional from time to time."

B. started crying quietly. Dr. Goldstein waited until she stopped. "Any new symptoms?" he asked me.

I told him about the sugary midnight snacks. Also that B. had begun closing doors—closing herself off in one room or another to take naps that went on for hours.

Dr. Goldstein was more worried about the closing of doors than the midnight snacks. "What feels better about being by yourself?" he asked.

Out of nowhere, B. laughed. "It's not always that I want to be by myself!" The doctor and I laughed, too. We knew what she meant. I could be a pretty intense guy. Sometimes she just wanted to get away from me.

"I'm going to start a gentle additional antidepressant— Lexapro," Dr. Goldstein told us. "It tightens things up a bit, maybe makes you less vulnerable to wanting to isolate." He paused. "If I met you five years ago, would you have been some-one who preferred closing the door?"

B. shook her head. "No," she said quietly.

The immediate goal, Dr. Goldstein explained, was to get B. to be less "isolating" and less tearful. She should be sure she took her Aricept—the drug that specifically addressed her short-term memory loss. That was the one she needed to take for three months, consistently, before she could enter the clini-cal trial for the new insulin-based drug.

"The sweet tooth," Goldstein asked. "Any reflections on that?"

"I'm going to try not to have those things," B. said sheepishly.

"We want you to enjoy things, have pleasures," Dr. Goldstein said. "We just want to be sure it doesn't become a compulsion."

B. sat quietly, on the verge of tears again.

"Talk to the doctor, honey," I told her. "What do you feel?"

B. cried again.

"She's a little embarrassed," I explained to Dr. Goldstein, "because she's always bedazzled everyone, cooked, come out, smiled; now she has to think about . . . everything. It's tough."

"It's unsettling and dispiriting, I know," Dr. Goldstein said. He smiled sympathetically. "All the more reason we have to restore some of your confidence."

Easier said than done.

For this job of caregiver, which I hadn't signed up for, hadn't bargained on, never anticipated, I was doing my best. But my best wasn't good enough, not if I flared at the wife I loved who couldn't help herself. So that made me feel even worse: not just frazzled and tired and very depressed but *guilty*.

Since then I've learned that that's all too common among Alzheimer's caregivers, even the millions who are better at it than I am. Even the Mother Teresas! You're human. You can't help snapping sometimes when your loved one loses her handbag for the third time that morning, or asks you the same question again and again. It's just human to get annoyed. Counterintuitive as it seems, the trick is to care for yourself first. Take the time off you need, get a good night's sleep, let yourself have a little fun for a change. And when a friend offers to sit with your loved one for an evening, and bring over a home-cooked meal, don't be the martyr who says, "No thanks," to that. Your answer is: hell, yes.

In this "mild-stage" world we were in, neither B. nor I thought we needed a health-care worker coming into our home. B. was adamant: she didn't want anyone underfoot and in her personal space. She certainly didn't want someone telling her what to wear and how to cook! A couple of times, we did try bringing someone in on a very part-time basis, and found that he or she showed a little too much interest in our personal lives. Maybe they were just trying to be helpful, not getting nosy about a woman who had had her fair share of celebrity. But I was wary.

As for friends pitching in, that just never turned out well. Real friends had busy lives, and for all their earnest intent, they backed off after a time or two. New friends—or, shall we say, acquaintances—simply couldn't be trusted, at least not by me. What if a "friend" borrowed money from B. while I was away? How would she remember to tell me about it, much less get it back? What if they hurt her or were unkind to her? The what-ifs were numerous. So we held off on bringing someone into our home, paid or unpaid.

Then, too, we'd always relied on each other. We were a small family—just the three of us with Dana, since B.'s parents and mine had all passed—and a very tight-knit one. We weren't accustomed to asking anyone for anything. We didn't appreciate yet that we were in a new world where the old rules didn't apply, and where pride and privacy would have to be put aside. We just kept on as we had, pretending life was unchanged—or not changed so very much. Which led to the night of the car chase.

Dana was managing the restaurant now, and doing a good

job, but no twenty-seven-year-old can keep a kitchen crew and waitstaff in line on her own, even a woman as blunt and tough as my daughter. You have to crack the whip—instill respect, even *fear*—and if that means firing the sous-chef who gives you attitude, you do it. That's for the big mean owner to do. So I was down there almost every night, at least for an hour or two. But I'll be honest, I was also escaping my caregiver role—without a backup—leaving B. in the apartment on Central Park South so I could grab a bit of the downtime I liked best: socializing with customers at the bar.

I may lose you here, but the fact of the matter is I really like bars—my own and a lot of others. I'm a social guy! I like chatting up people I find at the bar, buying the next round, sharing a few stories, a few laughs, some spirited debate. The television show *Cheers* said it all for me: the place "where everybody knows your name." For a lot of years our restaurant on Forty-Sixth Street was just like the one on *Cheers,* with regulars there every night. Even now, with B. there less often, it sometimes felt like that. B. loved all this, too, before the veil of Alzheimer's came down around her. Should I have stopped completely now that B. didn't spend as much time with customers at the bar as she once did?

Anyway, I was there that night, at our restaurant bar, talking up two female patrons when B. walked in unexpectedly. She fixed me with a look, came right over to me, and punched me hard on the arm. Then she turned on her heel and marched out.

I was stunned—and embarrassed. True, the two female patrons were attractive. True, I was enjoying their company. One might even say, as B. declared later, that I was flirting a bit. Guilty as charged. But this was no different than a thousand other nights at our restaurant. Talking up the clientele, even flirting with the clientele, is part of the business, as every bar owner knows. B. had done her share on those nights, too. We both understood that the bar was our stage, and the roles we played were audience entertainment, but it was all left behind at the door. In all our years together, B. had never been jealous of me, nor did she have any reason to be. All that had changed here was B.

By the time I'd made my apologies to the women and gotten outside, B. was around the corner and gone. As I reached Eighth Avenue, my jaw dropped: there she was, driving past me in a black Mercedes-Benz G-Wagen, scowling at me through the closed window as she floored the accelerator. Her mood was startling enough, but even more confounding was how she had our truck. I'd just parked it down the street at a meter, and the garage in our apartment building had access to only one set of keys—the ones I was holding in my hand. Something told me to go down to the space where I'd parked the truck. The truck was there! So whose truck was she driving?

ELEVEN

New York City

Spring 2014

I jumped into our truck and headed uptown, having lost B. in traffic. The G-Wagen mystery was solved when I screeched into our building's underground garage. There was the other black G-Wagen—some neighbor's—its hood still warm. Apparently B. had thought it was ours, as had the garage attendant. Thank God she hadn't smashed it up. But where was she? Not upstairs, as I quickly determined. Just gone.

I had a hunch that B. might be at the bar of the Ritz-Carlton hotel, just down Central Park South. It was a favorite of ours at the end of a working night. I found her there in a highly agitated state. As soon as she saw me, she dashed outside and started running—in heels—toward Columbus Circle. I ran after her, but lost her in the crowd—she was running that fast. At least her life was no longer at risk behind the wheel. Maybe blowing off steam was what she needed to do. So I gave up chasing her and went back in for a nightcap or two. I'm not proud of that decision, but then there's a lot that I'm not proud of in my caregiver role. I'll just say this: it's the hardest job I've ever had.

Eventually I left the Ritz-Carlton, went upstairs to an empty apartment, and trusted to fate. It was too soon to report B. as a missing person; I didn't know what else to do. At some point, hours later, I sensed B. sliding into the sheets beside me. I curled around her like I always do, and went back to sleep. When she woke up, she gave me a sunny if slightly groggy smile.

She had no memory of the night before.

N ot long after that, we made the decision to sell our New York City apartment, with its wonderful thirty-fifth-floor view of Central Park, and move out to Sag Harbor full-time. We were agreed on that, for different reasons. I felt the city was becoming an unsafe place for B. I kept imagining strangers walking up to her on the street, recognizing her, hassling her, maybe even endangering her. Then, too, I didn't trust her driving in the city. Anything could happen. Out in Sag Harbor, she could drive into town on quiet streets, not have taxis and panel vans veering in front of her.

It wasn't a hard sell. B.'s city life had shrunk mostly to the apartment and walking Bishop in the park. She felt she'd be happier in Sag Harbor, and maybe she would. In the back of my mind, I worried that we might be doing a geographic, as they say in Alcoholics Anonymous: making a physical move with the hope of leaving the bad stuff behind. The bad stuff of Alzheimer's wasn't going to be left behind any more than moving will solve an addiction. But at least she'd be safe, in a beautiful setting.

The plan was a bit sketchy, but I figured I would come into Manhattan a day or two a week, do some business with our B. Smith licensees, and stop by the restaurant to shake the staff into shape.

We had decided, back in February, to go public by writing a book. We didn't know where it would lead, but it felt like the right thing to do. So far, it was still a private undertaking: just us starting to write down what happened each day, and trying to make it a story that would resonate, both for those fighting their own Alzheimer's wars—and for all those who knew and loved B. It was in June, as we were emptying the apartment and moving to Sag Harbor for good, that we took what felt like a much bigger step: coming out on television with the news of B.'s condition.

As it turned out, the *CBS Sunday Morning* show had been running a series called "The Longest Journey," on the impact of Alzheimer's on a growing number of older Americans. The host was Dr. Jon LaPook, who made us feel comfortable right away when he came to Sag Harbor with his crew.

B. was in the kitchen heating water for tea as the interview began. Not surprisingly, Dr. LaPook asked B. about cooking. "Do you remember the first dish you made?"

"Um, pineapple upside-down cake," B. said. "I was probably about ten years old."

For anyone in his television audience who didn't know B. yet, Dr. LaPook mentioned her triumphs in the food and life-style category. "Some even thought she was on her way to becoming another Martha Stewart."

That wasn't the first time B. had been compared to Martha Stewart, and it wouldn't be the last. We had mixed feelings about the comparison, but the truth was that both women excelled in the business of gracious living.

Gently, Dr. LaPook made his audience aware of where B. was at now. "Do you know the date today?" he asked her.

"No."

"Do you know the month?"

"No."

"How about the year?"

"No."

"And what does that feel like?"

"I feel like crying," B. said. "Things like that make me very sad."

For the segment, Dr. LaPook interviewed Dr. Martin Goldstein at Mount Sinai. "We typically see Alzheimer's as a disease of old age, of frail, weak people near the ends of their lives," Dr. Goldstein said. "That's not B. B. is bright, dynamic, active, energetic, engaged, eloquent. B. sharing her story can change the game in terms of how people see Alzheimer's."

The show's producers wanted to know how I felt about B. getting Alzheimer's. "She has it. We have it. We have to deal with it," I said. "More people are going to have it. And you know what? If you don't talk about it, you're not going to make a difference."

"Even with Alzheimer's, I think that things are going to work out," B. added as the piece ended. "I'm going to do my best to make it work out for me, and for as many people that I can possibly help, too."

That got me. "I love you," I said.

"I love you, too," B. said. "I'm lucky to have you as my husband and best friend."

"I'm lucky to have you, too."

LESSONS LEARNED

Keeping Track of the Meds

Many well-functioning people in their sixties take a number of pills daily for various needs. Even with clear brains, they have to focus on getting the mix right. For a patient with early-stage Alzheimer's, that soon becomes a daunting challenge. Yet, out of pride, mild-stage patients often insist on handling their drugs themselves—the way B. did. When they lose track of which drug to take when, they may give up and put the vials in some hiding place to deal with at a later time. Often, they forget where they hid them. Sometimes, as the disease worsens, they mistake their pills for candy.

In our household, pill confusion and loss caused a lot of WTF moments until Dana intervened. She kept the pills in a place only she knew; dispensed the pills herself; and watched to be sure that B. actually swallowed them.

A better solution, at least for the early stages, is a high-tech pill dispenser. Like a home-alarm system, it's linked to a central office. When too few or too many pills are taken, an email or call is prompted. But for this to work, the dispenser has to be properly filled by the caregiver.

Ultimately, as the disease progresses, a home health-care worker is the best one to handle the allocation and administration of all drugs. But of course, that presumes a family dealing with Alzheimer's can afford a health-care worker. Not all can.

Hallucinations

B.'s occasional sightings of shadowy figures in a corner of the room is an all-too-typical symptom among Alzheimer's patients. Sometimes hallucinations arise from a patient's need to make sense of a situation: a deliveryman she didn't expect becomes a marauder. Often, a drug seems to provoke them: in B.'s case, the antidepressant Wellbutrin led directly to hallucinations, especially when overused; when the drug was removed from her daily intake, the hallucinations went away. Unfortunately, just removing or changing a patient's drug regimen may not do the trick. If hallucinations persist, they may indicate increasing brain damage.

At that point, of course, a doctor should be consulted. But a caregiver can at least avoid exacerbating the situation by telling the patient that what she's seeing isn't real. That will only upset her further, since what she sees is real to her. Better to offer a soothing response: "I don't see that, but I'm sorry you do." Then, if possible, ease her into a different room or out for an errand; upon her return, with any luck, the hallucination will be gone.

Profanity

As Paula Spencer Scott notes in *Surviving Alzheimer's*, a person never known for swearing is not now doing so by coincidence. It's a new behavior, brought on by Alzheimer's. "In dementia . . . there's damage to the part of the brain's processing centers involved in self-control," Spencer observes. "The person becomes less able to regulate certain behaviors, including language." Some Alzheimer's patients will belch or pass gas loudly:

the same mental governor on those actions, acquired in child-hood, is no longer at work.

Gently asking the patient to refrain from harsh language or insults may work; if not, ignoring the language may help you both.

Often, this behavior is brought on by frustration on the patient's part about something else altogether. Perhaps children at the table are talking too quickly for the patient to understand them; perhaps your talking on the phone stokes fears in your loved one that you are making arrangements to have her placed in an assisted-living home. Perhaps bathing or dressing has grown too daunting, and the loved one is venting in response. In B.'s case, I haven't yet figured out what the trigger might be; fortunately, she hasn't had too many episodes of profanity, and at the end of the day, given everything else we have to worry about, profanity is pretty far down the list. I mean, what the fuck, right?

CAREGIVER GUILT

Why does a caregiver who devotes so much of his time to a family member with Alzheimer's always end up steeped in guilt?

For me, the guilt came, at the start, from letting my frustrations get the better of me. I adore my wife but I would lose my patience when she forgot what I told her an hour before. I knew I shouldn't hold her to the standard of a healthy person, but I did—and felt guilty for that.

That's one kind of guilt. Another is the guilt a caregiver feels at taking time for himself. When I feel the need to get away from B. for an hour or two—perhaps to meet a friend for drinks—I'm taking the guiltiest of pleasures. How dare I have any fun while B. is at home in a cloud of confusion?

At least I love my wife. Some caregivers struggle with the guilt of having conflicted feelings about the family member they're tending: the spouse they no longer love as they once did; the parent, perhaps, who never stopped being hypercritical. The caregiver may resent the role fate has sentenced him to— and then feel guilty about *that*.

A loved one's worsening condition stirs more guilt. If only the caregiver had done more! The prospect of putting her in a nursing home? That stirs guilt, too, especially if the loved one ever made the caregiver promise not to do so.

Guilt is, to some extent, unavoidable: it goes with the territory. One way to temper it is not to set the bar as a caretaker too high. Don't feel you have to be perfect! And don't punish yourself when you fall short of that self-imposed standard. Aim to be a pretty good caregiver, not a perfect one: B-plus is good enough. Heck, B-minus is just fine. The goal isn't to do everything right. It's to keep your household from falling apart. Pass/fail—that's the standard I've learned to go by.

Navigating Emotional Land Mines

Caring for a loved one with Alzheimer's is trying enough to make anyone feel like taking the "loved" out of "loved one" on a regular basis. It's maddening—so much so that what caregivers tend to feel more than anything else is anger. I should know— I've had more blowups with B. than I could possibly count. But over the time it's taken to write this book, I've done a better job of keeping my frustrations in check—enough even to offer a few thoughts to others going through this slow-motion ordeal.

ANGER

Anger *is* understandable. But it's damaging to both caregiver and patient. If a person with Alzheimer's insists on eating with his fingers, admonishing him to eat with a knife and fork will do no good. It won't correct the way he's eating; it will upset him and make him anxious, and it certainly will upset the caregiver. Correcting the loved one as if he's rational is, itself, irrational. Letting the loved one's behavior stir anger is irrational, too.

One instinct is to tamp down one's frustrations and pretend they'll go away. Another is to blow one's stack. Better to try a middle course: recognizing the reality that your loved one has Alzheimer's and can't control herself, and just letting that anger go.

This is easier said than done. But for a caregiver, even changing the language he uses to express his feelings can start to temper them. In *Coping with Alzheimer's: A Caregiver's Emotional Survival Guide,* Rose Oliver and Frances A. Bock advise cutting out "must" and "should"—as in "he must stop eating like that," or "she should stop acting like that with me." Instead try "I would prefer that she not do that, but she might anyway."

Instead of "She ruined my life," try "My life has been changed as a result of her illness. So has hers. That's our reality."

Instead of anger, try channeling your feelings into disappointment and acceptance. As Oliver and Bock put it, "Why let the patient control your emotions?"

Guilt and anger lead, inevitably, to resentment. A caregiver resents the loved one who got sick and took over his life. If members of his family aren't doing their share, he will all but certainly resent them for that. Just as likely, he resents friends who get to live the happy life he led himself, before Alzheimer's knocked on the door.

Support Groups

These dark, grim sentiments go with the territory. But they can be confronted. Start by admitting them, and letting them out in constructive circumstances: with relatives, good friends, or, better yet, a support group where you can hear others vent, too. The one person to avoid sharing those dark feelings with is the patient. She can't help being in her situation any more than you can help being there with her. Anger and resentment directed at her will only upset her and exacerbate the traits that are driving you crazy as it is.

So, about caregiver support groups? I'll be honest: I haven't attended a support group yet myself. I did look online for one out here in the Hamptons, but there wasn't one nearby, and driving nearly an hour to get to one, while leaving B. at home, seemed counterproductive. There was no shortage of support groups in Manhattan, but that meant, of course, an even longer commute, now that we were in Sag Harbor—committing most of the day, in fact. This is a case, I would suggest, of do what I say, not what I do. I know that support groups can be enormously helpful. Not only do they give you perspective and insights on your day-to-day challenges as a caregiver; they also put you in touch with resources, from the local branch of the Alzheimer's Association to homegrown groups. I hope you find one near enough to attend. As our own situation progresses, I have no doubt I'll seek one out. For now, I'm relying on my doctors, my friends, and the occasional Dark 'n Stormy to take the edge off.

THE TRAP OF SELF-PITY

I'm the first to admit I feel sorry not just for B., but myself. No doubt about it, I've been dealt a rough hand.

B., of course, has been dealt a worse hand! So has your loved one. Focusing on that is one way to keep the self-pity in check. It also helps to be clear-eyed about your situation. It's bad, all right. Really bad. But are you going to get through it? Yes. I can't tell you how many times I've said, "I can't stand this . . . I can't go on . . . This is more than I can bear." But I *am* standing it, I *can* go on, and as hard as it is, it's *not* more than I can bear.

The point, as Oliver and Bock observe in *Coping with Alzheimer's,* is that caregivers have the power to put a more positive spin on the thankless task they've drawn—one that makes them feel less miserable while they're doing it. Instead of "I can't stand this" or "I can't believe it," try "I wish this weren't our situation, but it is, so there we are." Practice makes . . . not perfect, but less painful.

This isn't intolerable. It's sad and challenging but ultimately bearable. That's the emotional choice the caregiver can make. It's his loved one who has no choice.

PART 4

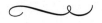

QUEEN OF THE
THREE RIVERS

That night when I drove down to find Dan at the restaurant—
it's hazy now. I was very angry at him. I just had a feeling
he'd be there talking to a woman, and so I wanted to check
it out. In the church next door to the restaurant, there was a show
at that time, called Cougar, the Musical, and every night when it
was over, the actresses would come in for discounted drinks. They
would bring theatergoers from the show with them, and everyone would get pretty raucous. It was good for business, but Dan
seemed a little too happy about it for my taste. So I was thinking
about that when I went to the restaurant. And there he was at the
bar, with a woman on each side!

I remember confronting him, and punching him in the arm,
then leaving to go to the bar at the Ritz—I've known Norm, the
bartender, for years. Then Dan came in, and I was still angry at
him, so I just left. I'm not sure where I went after that. I just
needed to blow off some steam. That's the way I am. If something
upsets me, I'll just take off.

I've always been an emotional person, but it's different now.
Sometimes my emotions overwhelm me now; maybe that's why I
like being alone.

When Dan is good he's very good—as a partner, as a dad, as

a friend to other people. He can be a tough boss, but also a very loving boss. He should have been in the military! It's who he is— which is okay. I'm pretty strong, too. Now that I have Alzheimer's, he wants to take care of me, but sometimes he makes me crazy. I feel like he's on top of me, asking if I want lunch before I know I'm hungry! Telling me what to wear and what not to wear, as if I couldn't get dressed myself. If I don't tell him I'm taking Bishop for a walk on the beach, he gets angry when I get back, like I've done something wrong. Some days it feels like everything I do is wrong by him. So I get mad, and he gets mad, and we argue in a way we never used to before. Which is silly. Are we going to change each other at this point? I don't think so. And does it matter? I mean, I'm not going anywhere; he's not going anywhere. We're in this for keeps, so we might as well be happy as much as we can.

Physically, I don't feel worse. The left side of my face still tingles—that's the one real physical effect of Alzheimer's for me. It feels like I got punched. It's like pins and needles. I'm not sure it's a side effect. It's like wearing a Spider-Man net on my face! It lasts all day. So far, none of the doctors has been able to explain that. It's not a typical Alzheimer's symptom. It's sure there, though, every day.

One thing I'm having trouble with these days is my handbag. I keep misplacing it. I'll put it down in my closet somewhere, and then the next day I can't remember where I left it. Or I go down to the basement to get something, and somehow forget it down there. Dan gets exasperated with me. I get exasperated, too! But what am I supposed to do? I think I'm going to remember where it is, and then I just don't.

TWELVE

SAG HARBOR

Summer 2014

That handbag drives me crazy.

It's a gold-sequined bag, big enough to hold all the essentials: change purse, cosmetics, identification. The kind of bag that everything gets dumped into, with no compartments, so that car keys get mixed in with old Life Savers, good jewelry, perfume samples, and spare change.

When her memory began to fade, B. would misplace the bag—either in the apartment or at the restaurant—and so the scavenger hunt would begin. I looked in the obvious places: dresser drawers, under the bed, in the bathroom. Dana was the one who realized that B. tended to put her bag in eye-level places. Like in the broiler over the stove, or on a hook in the coat closet. Or, at the restaurant, among the bottles over the bar. So we learned how to find it most days. Now that we're out in Sag Harbor full-time, B. has a whole new network of hiding places. Whether she means to hide her bag and other items, or just forgets where she's put them, I can't say for sure—and perhaps neither can she. But it's like a scavenger hunt every day here.

Always, when she gets ready for bed, B. takes the handbag into her closet. This is where it goes off the radar. The closet is more of a mess than ever. Now she balls up her clothes from the day and throws them in a pile, or sorts and re-sorts them by some foggy logic that will change the very next day. Hidden in those piles, a different pile each night, is the gold-sequined bag. B. won't let me look for it there: I'm not allowed in. Hours the next morning are spent looking for the bag, until B. re-emerges, triumphant. If I were a better caregiver than I am, I would clap and congratulate her. Instead I find it hard to hide my exasperation.

Over the last months, the gold handbag has grown heavier, as more and more spare change accumulates in it. B. never used to keep spare change in her bag. She does now. I'd guess that bag has come to weigh five pounds, getting heavier all the time. Kind of a metaphor, right?

The latest way B. deals with the bag is to carry it from room to room, morning to night. At least she tends not to lose it by day. But she won't let me empty it of all that spare change. It just clinks around with her, like a sack of gold, ready for purchases she no longer makes.

There is, I'm convinced, another reason why B. keeps that bag at hand. As tired as it's come to look, it represents her sense of decorum. Her mother always told her: a lady carries a bag. It holds your lipstick, your compact, your travel flask of perfume, and of course your mad money, enough to get you home if you and your gentleman caller get mad at each other. The fact that B. carries hers from room to room is not, to her, a sign of illness. It's proving she's still the kind of lady her momma taught her to be.

I get that, and I find it as sweet as you probably do. I just wish that her valuable jewelry hadn't found its way into that bag, never to be seen again. I'm talking a *lot* of valuable jewelry, six figures' worth. We had matching Rolex watches, even. No longer: hers is gone.

Possibly—and this is hardly reassuring—that missing jewelry may never have found its way into her handbag at all. B. may have tucked a bracelet or necklace into a balled-up cashmere sweater that went out for dry-cleaning—very expensive dry-cleaning. She may have put the odd piece or two into some kind of container that got mistaken for trash. All I know is that her beautiful pieces are gone, along with the life they symbolized. I could go out and buy her some new jewelry, but why? We'd both just worry about losing it—me a bit more than B. We've got enough stress without that.

The other day B. lost her phone. We called her number to no avail. It's probably in that closet somewhere, its charge depleted. B. calls almost no one now, and when friends call her, she fails to call them back. But we'll get a new phone—everyone has a phone, right? Perhaps the old one will surface first.

Meanwhile, B. spends hours each morning rummaging through her clothes. I used to think she was just looking for what to wear that day, and maybe she is, but it's more than that: it's an obsessive behavior. Unfortunately, that's part of Alzheimer's, too.

Let's give some of those clothes away, I say to B. She doesn't need five long summer gowns. I don't say this, but it's true: B. isn't likely to attend many fancy benefit dinners from now on.

Those days are gone. Let's give the gowns away, along with some of the older clothes she never wears; buy some casual clothes for the country home we now live in full-time. B. is adamant: no way. "I don't want new clothes!" she says. "I don't want fashion help!" Alzheimer's has touched whatever part of her brain governs shopping. She used to love buying new clothes. Now, she says, she wants no new stuff—only to keep what she has.

Actually, B. has a whole other wardrobe in storage—her Manhattan clothes. The sensible move would be to put a lot of the Sag Harbor clothes in storage with them, especially the winter wear, and bring some of the newer, summer-weight clothes out. But I can't make B. aware of that other wardrobe at all: out of sight, out of mind. And having me move *anything* out of that Sag Harbor closet is a no go with her.

Now the clothes closet drama has entered a new phase. B. is filling shopping bags with clothes and lining them up by the front door. She says she doesn't want to be a burden anymore to me. She also wants to be sure her clothes are safe from my meddling. So she's taking them home. What she means, as she explains every time she gets upset these days, is that she's taking them down to Everson, Pennsylvania, her hometown.

Every morning, B. goes out to her little Mercedes-Benz two-seater. It's a car I bought her some years ago as a present. Some hesitation or fear, or maybe confusion, keeps her from putting the bags in the car. Instead she get in and sits there, keys in hand, not quite up to starting the engine. And there she remains, until I come out and tell her it's time for breakfast.

THIRTEEN

EVERSON, PENNSYLVANIA

1949–1967

B. is one of Everson's best-known native daughters. Don't take my word for it: Google the town, and up she pops. They're proud of her there, but that pride came later. Growing up black in a white working-class town was a challenge, to say the least.

Everson was, and is, a largely Polish and Italian town, whose first immigrant settlers worked the coal mines. Of its nine hundred or so souls, perhaps fifty were African American. A lot of those were related to one another, by marriage if not by blood. B.'s father, Bill, served as a first lieutenant in the army in World War II, a trial by fire, for sure: first lieutenants led frontline troops and were killed in disproportionate numbers, black first lieutenants more so. Bill survived, and came to Everson because his bride, Florence, had grown up there, and because there was work at the U.S. Steel mill in nearby Clairton.

Every morning, Bill and a few other local men would carpool to the mill. They wore plaid shirts and jeans, even in summer, and carried more clothes with them, because they worked at the battery, and without those clothes, they might get scalded or burned to death. Once they got to the mill, they put on the extra layers, along with protective helmets and face shields, and respirators so they didn't breathe in toxic fumes. Then they started their shifts at one of the most dangerous jobs in industrial America.

The battery was a two- or three-story structure containing lots of ovens into which crushed coal was poured. The coal's impurities were baked out, leaving pure coke, the ingredient that makes steel as strong as it is. Bill and the other battery workers tended those fires, so close that without their extra clothes, the heat would have burned their skin. Each oven had a manhole-like cover atop the battery with four holes; if the wrong lid was lifted with an industrial hook, flames would shoot out and incinerate anyone in the immediate vicinity. When the baking was done, a heavy metal door on either side of the battery was opened, and a big industrial ram pushed the purified coke onto the so-called hot car, which then rode up a track to the quenching tower, where water cooled the coke down, and out to the railcars waiting to take the coke to market. Bill operated the hot car, too.

To compensate for the risk, battery jobs paid better than any others at the mill. Still, not many men, Polish or African American, felt the extra money was worth the risk. Bill Smith did—and spent the greater part of his working life at the Clairton battery.

Bill would come back tired and grimy, but he didn't stay in his work clothes for long. He'd shower and change, and come into the big kitchen where Florence was cooking the family dinner. The kitchen was the heart of the Smiths' home, where everybody gathered. Bill would pick up his guitar and start singing jazz songs to entertain them all. He had a beautiful voice, and so did B.'s mother. So, in fact, does B. The first time she broke into song, I was stunned. It was pure, a clean sweet voice like her physical presence. She was a gospel-singing church angel, she really was.

She still is.

Both Bill and Florence were frugal, and with Bill's battery job wages, they managed to buy a two-family house at the edge of town, overlooking the railroad tracks and a pretty creek beyond. It had an ample backyard with apple and pear trees, along with a grape arbor. "It was a really big house," B.'s cousin Randy recalls. "It still is." Their own living space had a big eat-in kitchen, a dining room and antiques-filled living room, and two upstairs bedrooms, one for Bill and Florence, the other for B. Their three boys slept in the attic, but that was hardly a sacrifice, since Bill had made it into a dormitory with wood paneling that slid open to reveal shelves for each boy, and single beds, each with a dresser and lamp, all in a neat row.

Bill and his brother were both woodworkers: they made all the kitchen cabinets, too. Florence was the cook extraordinaire, making every meal from scratch, as her mother had done before her. She cooked classic southern dishes, from chitlins to pigs' feet to collard greens. From the apple trees out back, B.'s mother made wonderful apple pies. They kept a vegetable garden out back, too, and a lot of the family's food came from there. Like most small-town folk in and around the Appalachian foothills, they did a lot of canning for winter—tomatoes, especially. They'd also fill their Mason jars with apple jelly, heat the jars, and seal them tight. From their apples, they even made wine.

Decades later, B. still remembers her mother's kitchen clear as day, how hot it was when a pie was in the oven, or corn bread baking, and dinner cooking on top. By the age of twelve or thirteen, B. cooked a lot of those dinners herself for her family of six, because that's what children did: they pitched in. For B., the very essence of summer was sitting out on the back porch on an August evening after dinner with her family, drinking her mother's homemade root beer while her father serenaded her mother with his strumming. Life didn't get any better than that.

Along with cooking good dinners, B.'s mother filled the house with fresh flowers. On a Friday or Saturday night, she and Bill would dress up and head into town for a restaurant dinner. Both were stylish dressers—Bill in a dark suit, Florence in a sundress, both of them in hats. That was where B. got her first exposure to fashion.

The Smiths instilled strict church values in their four children. B.'s father was a Jehovah's Witness, her mother a Baptist. From early on, B. went door-to-door with her father selling copies of *Awake* and *The Watchtower.* It was hard work, but it taught her what selling was about: not being afraid of the stranger inside the door, and learning how to pour on the charm. "One thing about being a Jehovah's Witness," B. likes to say, "you learn to talk to people." Before long, B. was selling newspaper subscriptions and women's magazines. She was a budding entrepreneur.

The Smiths were a poor black family, so no one went to the doctor unless there was an emergency. Mostly, they took care of themselves. B. remembers her father giving himself insulin for his diabetes. Clearly he inherited the condition: all of his seven siblings had diabetes, too. Lois Smith, who married B.'s older brother Gary, confirms that a high incidence of diabetes runs in the family, and she should know: she worked for more than forty years as a hospital technician. She came into the family in 1968 and says that Bill died in 1978, as much from the heart problems brought on by diabetes as from the diabetes itself. She doesn't recall Bill having memory issues, but maybe that was just a function of time: Bill died at sixty, too young to enjoy his modest retirement savings from all those years working at the battery. Too young, perhaps, to get early-onset Alzheimer's, genetic as its legacy usually is. Or possibly Bill did have early-onset Alzheimer's, and the heart disease killed him before the Alzheimer's could. As I would soon learn, all these factors tend to crop up with African Americans of a certain age: diabetes, heart disease, hypertension, and Alzheimer's.

I never knew Bill, but I did spend time with B.'s mother, Florence, as sweet a soul as I have ever known, until her death in 1988. She, too, died of diabetes complications. To me, B.'s mother never seemed more than typically forgetful for a woman her age, but then, she passed young, too: seventy-four. Of B.'s three brothers, two are alive and apparently healthy, but Gary, the brother Lois Smith married, died, like his father, of diabetes, at fifty-five.

Not until B. was diagnosed did the question of how her parents died seem significant. For this poor black family from rural Pennsylvania, no paper trail exists to prove which of B.'s ancestors on either side, going back generations, had Alzheimer's before her, but B.'s condition suggests that some did. And her parents' stated causes of death on both sides—diabetes and heart disease—both now seem possible precursors to Alzheimer's disease. All we know for sure is that since B. has no natural children of her own, her own inherited Alzheimer's, if inherited it is, is a genetic pathway that stops with her.

Everson did have a few other black families, but no amount of churchgoing could sugarcoat the fact that there were social and racial ceilings. B. couldn't be a cheerleader in high school, or join the 4-H club. Black students just weren't welcome. Undeterred, B. started her own home economics club, and made herself president: she and her fellow club members cooked and sewed.

Everson wasn't the Deep South. B. worked as a candy striper at the local hospital where she was born. She had both white and black friends. Yet she couldn't be a model at the local department store, either. That was frustrating, because what B. wanted to do, above all, was model.

One day B. saw an ad in a Pittsburgh paper for the John Robert Powers modeling school. She looked into it, then went to her father, who was not only very religious, but very strict. Would he mind if she took a Saturday course there, paying her own way? Absolutely not, her father declared: modeling school sounded racy. B., her sales skills honed, was ready for that. "Actually," she told him, "it's also a finishing school." *Finishing school.* That sounded proper. Grudgingly, her father said yes.

At first, B. took the bus home late each Saturday afternoon from Pittsburgh, a ride of twenty stops, then babysat to earn the money to pay for her modeling supplies. When she graduated from high school, she moved into an aunt's apartment in Pittsburgh. She also started teaching modeling at the Powers school. So striking was she that she was named the city's first black Miss Triad, Queen of the Three Rivers.

One day at the hairdresser's—one of those hairdressers who worked from home and passed on the local gossip and news—B. heard about a family that needed a governess for their young daughter. The parents, it turned out, were caterers: they cooked passenger food for Allegheny Airlines. Under their tutelage, B. came to like catering as much as she liked modeling.

B. started going to New York City to audition for major modeling agencies. She'd wanted to live there ever since her parents brought her and her three brothers to the 1964 World's Fair. Her brothers couldn't have cared less about returning, but to B., New York was the shining city on the hill. She learned that the Ford Modeling Agency didn't accept black models. But Wilhelmina Cooper might. That was enough for B. At seventeen, she left home for New York City, set on making a life for herself.

FOURTEEN

Sag Harbor

Summer 2014

B. gets sort of childlike these days, I guess you could say. If I correct her, or ask if she's forgotten a plan we discussed just minutes ago, she'll break into tears. She feels a child's sense of shame, and guilt. Harsh words are spoken on either side, until we dribble into silence again.

Yet sometimes, just as I'm gripped by despair, a glimpse of the old B. shines through. The other day I couldn't think of someone's name, and I asked if she recalled it. She did! The fog can lift, and when it does, the intensity of those moments takes my breath away. We look at each other, and it's like she's in a rowboat at the end of a pier where I'm sitting, and we're close enough to touch. Then the tide starts to pull the rowboat away, and again the fog rolls in, until the boat disappears and there's only the sound of rowing, somewhere out there, past where I can see.

With B., time heals all wounds, emotional ones anyway. The healing process lasts maybe twenty minutes, an hour at most.

She forgets; the day goes on. I'm the one who remembers the fight, and nurses his hurt, even as I realize I have no cause to feel upset at all—not when she is going through what she is, and not when the wife inflicting it on me is someone else. No, that's not true: when she's my wife *and* someone else that this awful disease has created.

Along with that handbag, the mess is what gets me. Remember that Dr. Seuss book about Oobleck, the stuff that just gets everywhere? B.'s clothes and shoes, and yes, her bags and other belongings are like that. They spread from the closet across the living room and down into the basement. Sometimes I make her go down there with me and see what I'm talking about. "We have twenty comforters down here! Why six duvets? Why not give them to people who need them?"

I see now that these things began to accumulate four, maybe five years ago, along with the first, unnoticed symptoms of her disease. Some people with Alzheimer's become hoarders; I'd say B. is pretty close to being one herself now. They forget they bought a new comforter, say, and buy another each time they go shopping. Some hoarders collect items of no particular value: newspapers or magazines. They lose the capacity to judge what's worth saving and what should be thrown away. Sometimes they hide the items, afraid their treasures will be taken by their care-givers. For now I just try to contain my frustration, and when B. refuses to throw out those extra comforters, I give up after the first or second attempt to talk her around.

There *is* no talking her around. More and more I'm coming to terms with that. In some ways she's the same old B. In other ways that B. is almost gone. I've come to feel that Alzheimer's is like a tornado moving through a town. It destroys some buildings and leaves others untouched. You can thank God for the ones that were spared, or you can shake your fist at fate. As far as I'm concerned, it's the luck of the neurological draw, brain cell by brain cell, plaque by plaque.

Often, these scenes end a new way now. After one or two angry exchanges, B. just walks away. She goes into our room, or one of the guest rooms, and slams the door shut. That's even worse than arguing: it's the sound of one hand clapping. I want to engage; I want to resolve. But now the door is closed, and if I barge in, I'll just provoke a new round of angry accusations. So I let the door stay closed, and the hours pass. When she finally reappears, she's forgotten what led her there. Chances are she's cheerful again. Gently, I ask her what she does in that room with the closed door, hour after hour.

"I just like it," B. will say. "I like being alone."

This, too, is classic Alzheimer's behavior, I've learned. B. is retreating, not only from me but from everybody she knows. When Dana first came home, she noticed that B.'s phone message box was full. She had about forty missed calls and a whole lot of unanswered texts. Dana tried getting B. to call back some of those friends. B. refused to do it. When we brought it up with Dr. Goldstein and Dr. Gandy, they told us being sociable was like exercise for the brain—absolutely essential, especially for someone with Alzheimer's.

Who was better at socializing than B.? She'd built her brand by socializing. That was what she did, as well or better than anyone. No longer. The way Dana put it, back when we had our high apartment on Central Park South, is that B. had become like Rapunzel. Friends on the sidewalk thirty-five flights below wanted her to let down her hair, but B. just wouldn't do it. She's only more that way now. I think she's embarrassed because she knows she's different, and she sees the pity in her old friends' eyes. Maybe, too, the sheer effort of trying to follow a conversation is too much for her now. Rather than try to keep up, she just backs off.

One night long ago, I got up to go to the bathroom, walked right down the hallway and—BLAM! I ran right into the closed bathroom door. B. had gotten up sometime before me—and pulled the door shut as she came back to bed. That's a new twist in door closing. I started cursing, then just shut it down. It was futile to keep ranting and raging. Instead I went out on the deck in the dead of night and just listened to the water lapping the shore. When I'd calmed down, I came back to bed and looked at my wife in the near darkness. There she was, sound asleep, with Bishop snoring beside her. All I felt, at that moment, was love.

Another night we fell into a furious argument about her closet—the fiftieth closet argument. Finally I threw up my hands and took Bishop down to the beach for a moonlit walk. When I came back, the sliding glass door to the deck was locked. So was every door! I went around the house four or five times, knocking on the doors. Was she angry, and punishing me? Had she hurt herself? Or had she locked up the house and taken off?

Finally I went to the garage. Thank God both cars were there: no midnight drive to Everson, Pennsylvania. But now I was really worried. Had she closed some door in the dark and then banged into it hard? I went back out to the deck, debating which way to break into the house. Then I saw a distant figure down the beach. I'd gone one way; she'd gone the other, maybe to find me, maybe to get away from me.

All I knew is that when she got close, she gave me that dazzling B. Smith smile, and waved. And once again, my anger melted away.

Often these days, when incidents occur and I'm trying to keep my temper in check, I turn to the sanest one in the room: Bishop. If B. is venting, as she does tend to do now, I'll look at Bishop, and he'll look at me. It's almost as if he's saying "Just chill out, it's not that bad, you know she doesn't mean it."

I'll raise an eyebrow. Really, Bishop? You think this isn't so bad?

"That's right," Bishop's gaze will say. "I got challenges, too. And by the way, I want some more food."

FIFTEEN

NEW YORK CITY

Summer 2014

Last spring, when we sold the apartment on Central Park South, Dana had to find a place of her own. She found one in the Chelsea section of Manhattan: the studio from hell, as she calls it. The stripper bar Score's is down the street; so is the High Line, with its crowds of tourists. There's grinding, relentless noise until 4 a.m., and then at 7 a.m., construction starts next door. Dana works at the restaurant each night, gets back to her studio late, and puts the pillows over her ears. She would still be living in Washington, D.C., in an apartment she liked, with friends nearby, if not for her mother's Alzheimer's. She'd still have the job she liked, too, as catering manager of B. Smith's in D.C., if B. was well and we'd managed to do enough business at the Union Station restaurant to keep going. Alzheimer's has turned her whole life upside down.

I think B. knows and appreciates that Dana is at the New York restaurant each night. She knows Dana is living on her own again, too. She just can't remember the neighborhood, and she keeps thinking Dana is sharing her apartment with three or four other girls, as she did in college. Now that Dana is gone, I'm the keeper of the drugs again. I'm better at it than before. Used to be, with a thirty-day supply, we'd get to the sixth day and B. would have only twenty-one left, which meant she'd taken three extra pills. Now I've got that under control: the drugs stay on my side of the vanity, and I personally hand them to her each morning.

I guess if there's any good that's come from all this, it's seeing Dana step up to the challenge. Alzheimer's does that to every family: shows you who's in and who's out, whom you can depend on and who gives you a pass. So it seems especially unfair that fate has socked Dana with a second blow.

Since childhood, Dana knew that her birth mother, Jocelyn, was not to be counted on, and would, by her own choice, play an insignificant role in Dana's life. By the time Dana was a teenager, she understood that Jocelyn wasn't just flighty. She had serious issues with drugs and alcohol. Dana still saw Jocelyn, but not often. She hadn't talked with her for two weeks when she got the news that Jocelyn had killed herself.

Of the many things I love about my daughter, one is that she's really wise, and another is that she's tough. These have been hard weeks for Dana, coming to terms with her birth mother's death. Was it a "fuck you" to all of us? A cry for help unheard? Or just the ultimately irresponsible act of a woman who lost her way long ago? I don't know. I feel bad for her family, but angry, too, at how she left Dana, and how Dana has had to be even stronger than she's been this last year.

I know Dana regrets her mother's passing. A part of her life has fallen away. But she's clear on this: B. is her real mother. B. is the mother who cooked her dinner every night of her childhood and helped her with her homework. B. is the mother who's still alive, and sick, and needs all the help Dana can give her. Dana is there to provide it. I couldn't be prouder of her.

Quite honestly, Dana has become a caregiver to me as much as to her mother. By that I don't mean just helping out. She's my reality check. "I can't help it!" I'll say after raising my voice to tell B. she's forgotten something I told her an hour ago.

"What did you expect?" Dana will shoot back at me. "People don't *want* to forget things."

For months now, Dana has told me to hire some outside help: a trained caregiver who can come in at least two or three days a week. B. is the one who says no. Only she doesn't say no exactly; she's too smart for that. She says she isn't against having someone in to help. It just has to be the right person. I've come to realize that no one, in B.'s mind, can be the right person. That's the point. She feels guilty that I've given everything up to be her full-time caregiver. She packs those bags for the drive to Pennsylvania—the trip back home she never takes—because she says she wants to stop being a burden to me. But she won't accept a stranger in her home, doing whatever it is home health-care workers do: helping her dress, cooking her meals, maybe cleaning that clothes closet. What she really resists is someone invading her personal space. She has done so much, and done so well. Surely she's earned her privacy, right? Well, yes, she has—until now.

To be honest, I'm part of that problem. I, too, balk at calling in someone to help. Why? Because I think I can do it all myself.

Because I love my wife, and can't stand the thought of someone else caring for her. And maybe—this is a hard one to face—because my whole life, for these last twenty-two years, has been lived in relation to her. I don't mean just in the romantic sense. I'm the other half of the B. Smith brand; I'm the businessman behind it. That's who I am; it's what defines me.

So I keep on being the caregiver myself, with all the feelings that that entails: love, irritation, sympathy, impatience, exasperation, guilt, until I can't take it anymore. That's when I head down to the beach with Bishop, look at the bay—and scream. "I can't stand this!" I'll shout to no one. "I just can't stand this anymore." Sometimes I get down on my knees on the sand and just pray.

I fear that I won't be able to do this on my own. Yet I also fear that whomever I get in to help won't give B. the level of care I want her to have.

My biggest fear is that I may succumb to a heart attack, or get into a fatal car accident. Maybe the chances are slim, but these things do happen, and even if they don't, I've had multiple health challenges. Along with prostate cancer, I've had a hip replacement and will almost certainly need another. I've had two back surgeries, and despite that, I have a lot of pain. What if I'm gone? Who will protect my wife from strangers intent on preying on her?

Just the other day, I came back home to find two real estate agents at the door. B. was about to invite them in without the slightest idea about why they were there. They *said* they were there to check out the house for some client who'd taken a fancy to it and might make an unsolicited offer. At the least, if I hadn't showed up, B. would have started a back-and-forth I didn't want us to have. What if the next set of strangers are burglars, posing as real estate agents and casing the place? What if some psycho takes advantage of my absence and attacks my wife? How will B. know not to invite him in, much less be able to say later what happened?

These are the film loops that play in my head as I lie on the beach, until finally I pick myself up, shake off the sand, and tell Bishop it's time to go home.

SIXTEEN

NEW YORK CITY

Fall 2014

One day in October, we came into the city to take a next step in getting B.'s story out to the public: an appearance on *The Dr. Oz Show.* We got up at 7 a.m., which is rare now for B. I asked her if she knew where we were going today. She did! I guess I'd told her enough times that it stuck. That made us both feel good.

As we left for the studio, B. looked like a million bucks, in black pants and a short jacket and heels. She looked even better after the makeup crew did their usual thing. Honestly, you wouldn't have guessed she was a day over forty—and one damned beautiful forty-year-old woman at that.

The Dr. Oz Show is what they call live to tape: they try to film it without any redos. The live audience gave us a warm welcome, and then we all settled in to watch a short video clip that the show had made when visiting us out in Sag Harbor. B. was asked how she felt these days. "When you're used to doing a lot of things at one time it feels like the air has been taken out," she told the camera, "and you're not quite the lady you were."

"Anyone who thinks this is a walk in the park—it's not," I said to the interviewer. "You're expecting what you had, but you don't have what you had. But you still have her."

Then the lights came up and the crowd gave us a hand, and Dr. Oz started asking us questions. He wanted to know how B. was feeling.

"I feel very good," B. said. "I have been working out a little bit, cooking a little bit, doing things with the family and the family dog. Trying to keep our life going forward on the same plane that it always has been."

"She has always been very independent," I chimed in, "a person who figures out how to do things regardless. She could wear a gown, go downstairs, cook, sing, and go upstairs. She was gracious and you knew it wasn't a façade."

Dr. Oz asked a question I was hoping he'd ask. "Why do African Americans have twice the incidence of Alzheimer's?"

"More diabetes, more heart disease—and they're hesitant to get help," I replied. That was an issue I planned to beat a lot more loudly as this journey unfolded.

When the interview was over, B. stayed and interacted with the audience. An elderly Italian lady came up and embraced her, kissing her again and again. Dr. Oz and I shared a look, and laughed. I knew what he was thinking. It was what I was thinking, too. You can't fake the warmth that B. has about people, even people she's never met before. And they can sense that right away.

Being out in Sag Harbor on our own, it's easy to forget how many people love B., but they do. Oh boy, do they. Soon we would learn just how much.

LESSONS LEARNED

Rummaging

B.'s daily sorting through her clothes closet is the most common form of what Alzheimer's counselors call rummaging. It can happen with silverware and kitchen goods, garages full of tools, and basements full of bric-a-brac. The rummager rarely finds what he may have started looking for; the rummaging becomes an end in itself: repetitive behavior that may arise from boredom, lack of exercise, vulnerability, or a need to feel useful.

Not infrequently, rummaging can lead to hoarding. The person with Alzheimer's may start collecting old newspapers or magazines—month after month after month—or start hiding something of value, like the jewelry that I gave B. Unfortunately, hoarders may forget their hiding places.

In *Surviving Alzheimer's,* Paula Spencer Scott suggests looking for "triggers." "Does the behavior begin or increase when your loved one is tired or in the company of new people? Is there too much background noise? Could it be related to being left alone or not having anything to do?"

Acceptance is the best approach—with an eye toward what, perhaps, the rummager is expressing on a deeper level by her actions. There is, after all, nothing harmful about rummaging or hoarding, unless something dangerous like guns or sharp knives is involved. Hugs and love can provide the assurance a person with Alzheimer's needs to break the pattern; finding a more constructive task for the person to do can also help. The fact is, most patients with Alzheimer's just want to be useful, as they once were.

If the behavior persists, a caregiver may want to consider moving the objects: driving those old newspapers and magazines to the dump. I've found with B. that that can break the cycle.

B.'s ever-accumulating piles of clothes in her closet have finally driven me to action. I couldn't bring myself to tell the sort of white lie that caregivers often do: removing the objects in question when the patient is asleep, and later reporting they're in storage somewhere. Instead I've managed to persuade her to put a lot of her clothes in storage—for real—and I take her with me when I bring them to the storage unit.

Going Home

At first, B.'s talk of going home to Everson, Pennsylvania, both startled and hurt me. B.'s parents were long dead. So was one of her three brothers; a second lived in Texas, while the third, who did live in Everson, had not been close with B. for years. Aside from her late brother's wife, and her cousin Randy, she had almost no one to visit down there. Gradually, I came to see that "going home" is more a state of mind for B. than a physical place. So jarring and disruptive is Alzheimer's that patients often long for the place where they remember being happy and confident, where life seemed to stretch on forever. That B. had few family members to visit left may not have entered her mind.

As with all behavioral changes that come with Alzheimer's, a caregiver should look for what might be the "trigger" for the yen to "go home." Maybe the patient feels disoriented by a new home or day care center. Possibly she feels anxious and depressed—and home, not surprisingly, seems the antidote to all those dark feelings. A caregiver's first reaction is usually to use reason. "This *is* your home," he may say. But reason plays no part in these disease-provoked behaviors.

You could try to take the patient on a short drive, perhaps for a restaurant meal, then declare, upon returning, "We're home!" Another idea is to break out old photograph albums and let the loved one connect visually with her sense of home. Paula Spencer Scott has pretty unsentimental advice for the more ambitious caregiver. "Don't bend over backward making a 'Trip to Bountiful' reunion visit to a home place," she writes. "Remember, someone with dementia rarely means home literally. . . . While such a trip can be fun (if she's physically capable), you have to brace for the possibility that even a visit to an intact old home won't satisfy the longing that's been expressed. If the place is gone or altered, even if your loved one can remember it, she may be even more confused."

EMOTIONAL UPS AND DOWNS

These are very common as incidents of forgetfulness grow more noticeable and severe. A task that becomes challenging, with too many steps—like cooking—may overwhelm the patient and lead to upset or anger: what doctors call a catastrophic reaction, because it's disproportionate to the situation at hand. Flare-ups and crying jags may just seem signs of a new irritation with one's spouse, as they did with B. and me. A related disorder, pseudobulbar affect (PBA), sometime tied to Alzheimer's, sometimes to a stroke or head injury, may provoke racking sobs intermittently all day.

The sooner these outbursts can be recognized as disease symptoms, the better. An aware caregiver can try to avoid "trigger" situations: assisting with tasks that have grown complex, helping the loved one complete a point in conversation, above all remaining gentle, and patient. A soothing tone works wonders; a shoulder rub never hurts. One caregiver in Paula Spencer Scott's book reported showing old comedy films every night, from Charlie Chaplin and Abbott and Costello to the Marx Brothers. "When my mother was laughing, she didn't cry. It was like turning the spigot off for a while."

CLOSING OFF FRIENDS

When B. closes doors, she isn't just pushing her family away. She's isolating herself from friends—in her case, quite a few very close friends she's had for decades. I do think she's self-conscious now, in a way she never was. She doesn't want to put herself in a situation where she can't keep up her end of the conversation. Nor does she want to see pity in the eyes of people who've loved and admired her for years. I think, too, that some of her friends aren't sure how to act, especially when B. fails to return a message. Should they assume she just forgot they called, and keep trying her, even at the risk of seeming intrusive? Or should they take her silence as a signal that she'd rather not talk to them now?

I'm not sure there's one simple answer. I do know B. has times now of wanting to be alone. I've also seen her listen to messages and decline to call back. Maybe in an hour she's forgotten that friend called, but her initial reaction is often to push that friend away—or so it seems.

To be perfectly honest, though, I may be part of the prob-

lem. I've got so much to juggle, between caretaking B. and trying to keep the business going, that I may not be as good a
message relayer as I should be. And maybe I should be pushing
B. harder to see her friends, even setting up social visits for her.

I do know this: along with diet and exercise, socializing
is one of the essential measures that doctors recommend for
anyone with Alzheimer's. One recent study of eight hundred
men and women, all seventy-five and older, showed that those
who were more active, physically and mentally—and more
socially engaged—were less likely to develop any form of dementia. Bridge clubs, dinner parties—and yes, for God's sake,
shuffleboard!

Or, for that matter, music. The other night I saw a very moving report on PBS about a retired businessman in his early seventies who has Alzheimer's. His memory is shot, but he hasn't
lost his chops at the piano. I mean, this guy can *play*. So once a
week or so, he joins a group of fellow musicians—all of them
impressive at their instruments, all of them struggling with
some form of dementia. Playing standards together makes them
happy; it may also be keeping their brains from deteriorating at
the rate they otherwise might. What really got me was the trio
of high school musicians who sit in with them—not out of pity,
or for extracurricular credit, but just for fun.

Here's the bottom line: a healthy diet and physical exercise
without social interaction on a regular basis won't be as effective in helping keep those brain cells alive.

PART 5

BRAVE, THEN
AND NOW

I have trouble remembering what Dan and I said an hour or two ago—it's true. But I remember Everson so clearly. We had a two-family house at the top of a hill at the edge of town—a steep enough hill that I had to walk my bike up it after I did my paper run, with all that money in my pocket to be divided: so much for the newspaper, the rest for me. One family rented the far side of the house, another family rented the basement. It was a big deal in Everson to own your own house, and have it be big enough for tenants. My parents got a lot of respect for that.

There was a back porch off the kitchen. From it, you looked down at the railroad tracks, and Joseph's Creek beyond. The trains would roar by at all hours of the night, like they were going through our kitchen, but we liked the sound—and that piercing whistle. I had a lot of trains, and train whistles, in my dreams.

We were always warned not to swim in Joseph's Creek; it might sweep us away. I don't know how likely that was: Joseph's Creek was pretty tame. Then again, none of us knew how to swim, none of my three brothers or me. So we stayed away from the creek. Instead, I liked to walk up the tracks, looking for berries. There was a lot more danger in that!

I was probably no more than eight years old when I started

going with my father door-to-door, selling The Watchtower. *My father was a great salesman. He had a wonderful smile, and when a door opened, he knew how to be friendly but not overly so: friendly but respectful. At some point, though, he changed his approach. Instead of knocking on the door himself, he stayed in the car and let me do the knocking. I'd be standing there, happy as could be as soon as the door opened, because I knew I was going to meet someone new. I'd start a conversation going, and at some point the person at the door would ask a question, and I'd say "Gosh, I'll bet my father can answer that." I'd give him a wave, and up he'd come, and soon enough we were inside, spreading the word. I remember my father giving out* Watchtowers *for whatever the people wanted to pay. I sold the Bibles—a lot of Bibles, to tell you the truth.*

My father and mother were a great couple. I never heard either one say a rude thing to the other. They never fought. They loved talking in the kitchen as my mother made dinner, eating out on the porch on summer evenings, and singing to my father's guitar.

Not long ago, my sister-in-law Lois sent it to me—my father's guitar. I took one look at it and burst into tears.

SEVENTEEN

SAG HARBOR

Summer 2014

Morning is the toughest time of day for us now. Will B. wake up happy, willing to follow the plan of the day? Will she dress herself in clothes that suit the weather? Most important, will she know where her handbag is? Or will this be . . . not a bad day, we don't call them bad days, we call them challenging days. On a challenging day, the handbag is missing, the car keys are gone, and the schedule is out the window.

On a good day, B. takes her morning pills without a fuss. We have breakfast, and we plan our day. We walk Bishop, I get in a few business calls, and then we go food shopping: the highlight of our day, or at least mine.

Before B. got sick, she loved food shopping. She loved to cook. She wrote three books on cooking and entertaining! All that's gone. I'm the one who gets us to the markets. I'm the one who insists we cook. I think all the choices intimidate B. now. She stops in the rice and pasta aisle, and for a moment her eyes dance at all the choices. Then she hesitates, and that look of uncertainty comes over her, until her eyes go dull and she purses her lips in a frown. I used to wait beside her, thinking I'd force her to make a decision, and that she'd feel better for that. As the seconds ticked by, my frustration would rise. I'd give her a choice: this brand or that? Eventually I learned to handle that moment—and so many others just like it—by saying, "How about this one?" I was making the choice for her, but that was what she wanted, too. In that sense, we were making it together.

At least, by the diet we stick to, we've never been healthier. We may even be keeping B.'s Alzheimer's from getting worse. That's the hope.

We've actually enjoyed the so-called Mediterranean diet. Fruit for breakfast, sometimes as a shake with wheatgrass and soy milk. Salad and vegetables for lunch, maybe an egg white omelet—and no refined carbohydrates! For dinner we eat cold-water fish like arctic char and black cod. And more vegetables, more salad, more protein. If we get hungry between meals, and need to snack, we'll have nuts instead of crackers or sweets.

Before Alzheimer's, B. did virtually all of the cooking. That was her choice; she liked it. She still cooks, sometimes, but it takes her longer. She doesn't follow recipes—she's always known how to put a dish together from what's available, and which herbs and spices will perk up a soup or stew. She still knows, but what starts as one dish may come out as another. She may start a salad for lunch, and presto! It ends up a smoothie. With kale and cucumbers and bananas, blackberries and blueberries. She just forgot what she set out to make, and started again halfway through.

Sometimes, just for fun, I'll give the Mediterranean diet a rest and shop for one of B.'s favorite dinners: dishes she came to know in Paris and Milan and Vienna as a top model traveling the world. Coq au vin, for one, veal schnitzel for another. Those tastes stir memories, and sometimes a story. Or dishes she loved as a child. One of her grandmothers had a chicken coop and introduced B. to chicken feet! Not long ago I saw chicken feet in the meat section of our local supermarket, and bought them on a whim, wondering if they'd stir childhood recollections. That night, as we cooked together, B. reminisced about Grandma Hart and all the meals she'd gotten from those chickens. There was a use for every part of the bird. Most of Grandma Hart's dinners came right from the backyard. I can't stand chicken feet myself, but I sure enjoyed the company. All those childhood memories are still vivid for B., unaffected by Alzheimer's—so far. As long as we stay back there in those early days, I can pretend she's the same old B.

We do that a lot these days: sift through those long-term memories. People say, "Don't dwell in the past." Let me tell you: with Alzheimer's, the past is the best place to dwell. You want to linger over every one of those sweet, long-ago scenes. They're where happiness still resides.

Other nights end in arguing—or worse. A few nights ago we met for dinner at the American Hotel. B. drove from the house, and I came in our other car from a business meeting. We had a nice dinner—and yes, a few drinks, even though I know Alzheimer's patients shouldn't drink; we just wanted to pretend things were normal—and then left to go home. I told B. to go first, in her car; I would follow. As soon as we rolled out of town, beyond the streetlamps, I saw that B. was driving with her headlights off. As she passed the little gas station not far from our house, a police car pulled out to follow. *Oh shit,* I thought.

B. pulled over, and I pulled over, too, maybe three hundred feet behind her. When you're a black man in America, you know exactly how a scene like this could turn out. A black man coming up the shoulder of the road, approaching a policeman in the dark?

"It's Dan Gasby," I called out. "That's B. Smith. She's on medication."

Fortunately, I knew the officer. More fortunately, he knew me. Instead of reacting defensively, he returned my greeting, and I went into my spiel about Barbara's condition and how her drugs disoriented her. It wasn't all that persuasive: Why was she driving at all if she was on that medication? Plus, there was the matter of the headlights, not to mention the alcohol on her breath, and mine. But we were less than a mile from our house, and the policeman just waved us home.

I knew we'd arrived at a destination I'd wanted to avoid, but could do so no longer. I made a private pledge that night not to let B. drive again. But in the interest of keeping a happy dinner from ending in anger, I said nothing about it to her. Instead, over a nightcap on the back deck, looking out at the bay, I steered us back to the past, to those early New York days when B. became a world-class model and all her dreams came true.

EIGHTEEN

NEW YORK CITY

1967–1985

I've tried to imagine how all alone B. must have felt as a young black model in New York City in the late 1960s and early '70s. She's told me the stories, but I can't quite grasp them. *No* black faces on mainstream fashion magazine covers. None inside those magazines, either. Not on the editorial pages, not in the ads. What would possess a seventeen-year-old black woman to come to New York—on her own—and go up against the entire white fashion world with nothing more than good looks and a smile? It takes courage, I'll tell you that. B. is the bravest person I know.

All too often, in those go-see days, B. would drop off her book—her big black book of modeling photographs—either at an agency or one of the fashion magazines. The receptionist wouldn't even try to hide her surprise. Back it would come, possibly opened, more likely not, with no word of encouragement from the unseen art directors beyond the reception area. Jerry and Eileen Ford simply didn't accept black models; other agencies took the same line, just not as blatantly.

B. did have one ally—a life-changing ally at that. Wilhelmina Cooper was a Dutch supermodel who with her husband had started her own agency—one with a unique approach. Wilhelmina had seen how easily models could be exploited, by unscrupulous men and employers alike. She wanted to keep her models safe. Instead of just getting them jobs, she managed their lives like a mother hen. Rene Russo was one of her future stars. So were Patti Hansen, Pam Dawber, and Connie Sellecca. Soon enough, they were not just B.'s fellow models, but her friends.

B. wasn't just invited in with open arms, though. Wilhelmina called her back three times, intrigued but wary. Finally she told B. to get new pictures done. B. met with a photographer the agency recommended, only to have him propose sleeping with her in return for printing pictures from the shoot. When this happened with another photographer, too, B. went back to Wilhelmina. "What should I do?" B. asked. "Can you help?" Wilhelmina took a drag from her extra-long cigarette with its holder and gave her a look that said, Clever you. B. wasn't trying to be clever. She was desperate. Wilhelmina was her last chance, and those sleazy photographers were keeping her from it. Wilhelmina must have heard that desperation in B.'s voice, because at Wilhelmina's direction, the agency set B. up with a hassle-free photographer, hair, and makeup—all at no cost. The moral to that story, B. would say years later in speeches: if you don't tell someone what you need, they can't help you.

Most of Wilhelmina's stable lived, on her orders, at the Webster Hall hotel for women on Thirty-Fourth Street: no men allowed above the first floor. B. took up residence there, too. To

her girls, Wilhelmina was more than a role model. She was their
surrogate mother. She wanted them to feel they were part of
her family; often, they did photo shoots up at Wilhelmina's big
house in Connecticut, and hung out there for hours afterward,
drinking and talking.

In her own way, Wilhelmina did what she could to break the
race barrier in modeling. One day she escorted B. and another
of her models to meet Dino De Laurentiis. The famous director
was conducting screen tests for his remake of *King Kong*. When
he saw B., he was stunned. Did Wilhelmina imagine a black
girl up there on the spire of the Empire State Building, doing
battle with King Kong? I remember asking B., "Why did you
go? Why even bother?" "Well," she said with that radiant smile,
"you never know!" The other girl Wilhelmina brought that day
did get the part: Jessica Lange.

At Wilhelmina's urging, B. began to take acting and singing
lessons. She worked up a nightclub act, and landed a gig at the
old Playboy Club across from the Plaza Hotel. She sang at another place called the Bushes, on the Upper West Side. At one
point she was in a reggae band as a backup singer with Debbie
Harry, before Debbie became Blondie. Another time she was in
a trio with two Freds—one of them future R&B king Freddie
Jackson. Sadly, the night that Wilhelmina was to come catch
B.'s act with Freddie, she had a stroke. B. kept looking at the
door, waiting for her to come in, until they got the news. Ever
after that, Wilhelmina's advice motivated B. "Do everything
you want to do," she told B. more than once. "Don't let anyone
stop you."

B. was—and is—a terrific singer. But modeling was her
forte. She became the first black woman on the cover of *Made-*

moiselle. She did cover after cover of *Essence*—no one before B. had had five *Essence* covers; they sold better on the newsstands than any other face. She did covers of *Ebony,* too. She could do young; she could do sophisticated. The only thing she couldn't do was white.

Magazine covers made her a star; commercials made her money. B. did more than one hundred television and radio campaigns. She sold Crest toothpaste with Lena Horne; she sold Colgate, too. She was the face of Pillsbury buttermilk biscuits, and Betty Crocker corn bread and corn muffin mix. She pitched Noxzema, USAir, Equal, Burger King, and many others. For all that success, though, B. never felt she had it made. Often as not, casting directors would find her too black. Others would say she didn't talk black enough. She had to fight for every job.

As she made more of her own money, B. rented an apartment and started decorating it with care. At the end of a modeling session she would ask the photographer if she could keep a prop or two: a fish tank, maybe, or a standing lamp. Usually the answer was yes. Finally, B. felt ready to invite some of the models over for dinner. The first dinner she gave was all ladies—gorgeous ladies—who oohed and aahed at all the hand-me-down objets. They wanted to know which photography shoot each one had come from. All were still struggling to make ends meet, as B. was, and they marveled at how resourceful she was. They saw, too, how naturally all those objets worked together. This girl from rural Pennsylvania had style! And cooked like a dream. None of the others ever entertained. Nearly every model B. knew ate almost nothing and never cooked, not even for themselves.

Why B. felt a need to host and cook dinners, she couldn't

quite say. Her mother's cooking, and those summer evenings of hungry, happy relatives and friends—that was part of it, for sure. Then, too, B. liked people. I mean she really liked people, virtually everyone she met. She just embraced new people with a pleasure they felt right away. I think, too, that the magazines she was appearing in now made a strong impression on her. There was glamour in entertaining. That was what those magazines conveyed. It was like entering another world. This was the world where B. wanted to live.

Often, after a downtown shoot, B. would come up to the East Side and have dinner alone in an elegant restaurant, just to experience, if only briefly, the dream of an affluent life. More than once, the waiters treated her rudely: they assumed she was a high-class hooker awaiting her john. Since modeling shoots were almost always during the daytime, she eventually got evening work as a restaurant hostess. She wanted to learn the restaurant business, for the inevitable time when she grew too old to model. One of her stops on that trail was a restaurant called America, on Eighteenth Street, a vast, high-ceilinged coliseum of a place, popular for serving huge portions of pasta in big white bowls. There B. worked her way up from evening hostess to manager.

Tragically, Wilhelmina died of lung cancer in 1980, at the age of forty. But B. was a big enough model now to survive that loss. She had changed her name from Barbara to B., and had all the shoots she could handle: the flip side of being a black fashion model was that once you made it, *everyone* knew you. She also had money, enough to consider opening a restaurant of her own.

NINETEEN

Sag Harbor

Fall 2014

It's October here in Sag Harbor, and the days are growing short. Over breakfast, B. will almost always ask me now: What should I do? I know she doesn't mean to add to the stress of getting through these days, but she does. I feel responsible for coming up with a daily agenda for her—and there just isn't that much to do, not when Alzheimer's has encased you in its fog. I know from reading some of the books on Alzheimer's that small, repetitive tasks can put a troubled mind at ease. I encourage B. to sort the coins she carries in that gold handbag. I get her loading and unloading the dishwasher. I know I sound like a prefeminist husband, but it pleases B. to be useful. Her favorite task is ironing: the sheets, pillowcases, and my shirts. She loves to see those linens and shirts military crisp. I keep my eye on that iron: I know that at some point, I'll have to take it from her, and there'll be no more ironing shirts. But as long as she can do it as well as she does, and as long as it pleases her, why not?

. . .

At our last office visit, our doctors, Sam Gandy and Martin Goldstein, told us new clinical trials were coming. B. would join at least one of those trials; we would take new pills and swallow another serving of hope. The problem is that B. hasn't yet logged enough consistent time on Aricept, the drug she needs to take first. She has to take Aricept for three months before she becomes eligible for a trial.

I no longer think, as I did just a few months ago, that B. can turn this disease around by joining a new drug trial tomorrow and popping the pill that makes her well. I know the odds. No panacea is coming next year to a pharmacy near you—not for those, like B., who are well into the early stages of Alzheimer's. The best hope we have for B. is a new drug that comes along soon enough to help alleviate her symptoms—better versions of the drugs we have now, which basically do nothing. Maybe in five years, other people in the mild stage will benefit from drugs that do more—drugs that "manage" the disease, as our doctors keep putting it, drugs that actually stop the disease from progressing. But how much these new drugs will "manage" Alzheimer's, and by when, are questions that our doctors, as nice as they are, seem unable to answer.

To be honest, our doctors at Mount Sinai haven't had much to tell us on any aspect of B.'s condition these last several months. She's taking her pills; they seem to be managing her moods pretty well, better than if she weren't on them; she hasn't stayed consistently enough on Aricept to be eligible for trials; and . . . that's about all the doctors have to say. It's like a gun went off and the race began, and B. and I started circling the track. But then everyone in the stands just sort of went home, and we're left going around and around with no one there to notice, much less tell us where the finish line is. We're just on our own, passing time: Alzheimer's time.

L ast week, at a friend's suggestion, I drove B. to a modest office in Southampton. Some Alzheimer's groups are just focused on drug research; others are just focused on care. The Alzheimer's Disease Resource Center (ADRC) has a foot in both camps. It's also the only go-to group for Alzheimer's on the east end of Long Island.

At the ADRC office, we met a broad-shouldered, forty-something woman with a booming voice and warm manner named Joan Motley, the office's outreach coordinator. For any of you as old as I am, she reminded me a bit of Jo Anne Worley on *Rowan and Martin's Laugh-In.* Joan heard me out for about half an hour and then held up a hand.

"Where do you think B. is now on the scale of the disease?" she asked.

"She's mild stage," I said, "but maybe it's progressed a little."

"I'm not hearing the 'early' anymore in what you're saying," Joan said. "I'm hearing the moderate. Within the three broad areas there are seven stages. I think you're in Stage Five."

"Stage Five, meaning what?"

With Stage Five, Joan explained, there is cognitive decline in the ability not just to remember, but to reason. "You're still rea-soning with B.," Joan said, "expecting *her* to reason. You need to look at this in a different way. B. no longer has that ability."

I felt bad having B. beside me, hearing such a blunt report. But what was to be gained by not telling her? Clearly, Joan had no hesitation about putting it out there.

"That's hard, I know," Joan said. "But it should take some of the weight off your shoulders. Because clearly you need help in caring for her—help for B., and time off for you."

Joan turned to B. "Are you still driving a car?"

B. nodded. "I think I should be driving more," she said with a little laugh, "but no one else thinks that. I've never had an accident. I drive to the store . . ."

Joan asked when B. had last driven.

"Actually about two months ago," I said. I told Joan about the scary moment that night after dinner at the American Hotel. "She has a tough time initiating things now. She'll get in the car but forget the key. She'll go back for the key and forget she went to get it."

"A lot of your perception has changed," Joan told B. "And that affects driving. Your reaction times are not as sharp. It's great you haven't had an accident, but it's no longer safe to go behind the wheel."

The stories I'd shared—of B. losing her handbag and having clothes all over her closet—were all too typical, Joan said. She turned to B. "You worry about where you put things: it's your stuff, what's dear to you, and you want to remain in control. But it's hard to keep track, and you get overwhelmed. You become a hoarder, not sure where anything is, but at least controlling the mess because it's your closet."

Now Joan turned back to me. "Dan, I'm going to speak very openly. You're coasting. We have to put on the brakes. You've been in denial, and denial keeps us from moving forward. The fact is, you've done a really good job of pulling this together. But now it's okay to get help. Until you do, your anger and frustration are just going to grow, and you'll be too burned-out to give B. the help she needs."

There was good news in this, Joan added, for both B. and me. Good news—right. Like it had been good news when B. was diagnosed with "mild-stage" Alzheimer's. *I'll tell you what good news is,* I thought. *You tell me a cure is around the corner. That's good news.* But I refrained from saying that.

The good news for me was that with home-care help on a regular basis, I'd have some downtime—time to recharge. B. would be able to do many of the things she'd stopped doing because they overwhelmed her. Like cooking. "That passion for cooking is not lost," Joan told her. "You just need someone next to you who can help. You'll feel relieved; you won't have to remember so much on your own."

But Joan didn't sugarcoat it. "Our challenges will become greater," she said to B. "Now is the time to start bringing in assistance, and getting you adjusted to someone other than your husband. There will never be a right time for you to take on someone. But you need to realize that for your safety, there's nothing but benefits in bringing someone in."

At that, B. started to cry.

"I know it's the pride," Joan said, more gently now. "And you want to do everything yourself. You're an extremely strong and confident person. But now it's hard to do everything. It's hard to invite a total stranger into your house, but you must."

"If it's the right person," B. said again.

"You can start off slowly," Joan said. "In particular, you want to target the days that Dan is in the city. There's a lot of hours in the day that B. is unsafe. If there was something on the stove, or a stranger at the door . . . B. just can't be left alone at home anymore."

I heard that; I took it in. She was right. It was time. We'd just have to see if B. could take it in and accept it, too.

LESSONS LEARNED

WHAT SHOULD I BE DOING?

Patients with Alzheimer's may be confused, but they know how sedentary they are. They wish they could be more active—and useful. Which is, of course, part of the longing to be who they were before Alzheimer's. Finding small tasks for them to do, as I do with B., is the best therapy you can practice. If there are tasks where the two of you can work together—all the better. So far, B. and I still cook together; those are probably B.'s happiest moments.

THE STAGES OF ALZHEIMER'S

Doctors refer to both a three- and seven-stage model for the progression of Alzheimer's. The three-stage model is, of course, simpler, but the seven-stage model allows for greater specificity on diagnostic tests. Here's the three-stage model:

Stage One: Mild/Early

Short-term memory loss becomes apparent, especially in regard to recent conversations and events. The patient may ask questions repeatedly, and struggle in speech to find common words. Writing may become difficult. Hand-to-eye coordination may become somewhat impaired: handling silverware at the table, for example, may be a challenge. All these symptoms may bring on, or be accompanied by, mood swings and depression and/or apathy. Driving may also be an issue. Generally, Stage One lasts two to four years.

Stage Two: Moderate/Middle

Long-term memory loss becomes evident now, too; childhood recollections may fade, and the patient may have trouble recognizing family members and other familiar faces. General difficulty understanding current events, confusion about time, and loss of awareness of place, even of one's own home. More dramatic mood swings and depressions, along with fits of anger and aggression; also uninhibited behavior. Sleeplessness is common; so is sleeping too much. Delusions may occur. Physical tremors and general slowness; difficulties in dressing and toileting. Generally, this stage lasts from two to ten years.

Stage Three: Severe/Late

Profound memory loss, inability to communicate and comprehend others. Needs round-the-clock help for all personal hygiene as well as to guard against falls. Issues with swallowing and incontinence. Delusions are common, even prevalent. At the end stage, the patient becomes immobile and unresponsive. Generally, it can last one to three years.

And here's the seven-stage model:

Stage One: No impairment; memory and cognitive abilities appear normal.

Stage Two: Minor, often unnoticed memory lapses; indistinguishable from the normal memory issues of aging.

Stage Three: More difficulty finding words; the patient often becomes aware of this before others do, and tries to cover it up. Objects often misplaced. New facts hard to retain. Some mood swings and depression.

Stage Four: Increasing short-term memory loss; difficulty in completing sequential tasks like cooking and driving. Planning becomes difficult if not impossible, as do simple mathematical challenges, like balancing a checkbook or just keeping track of loose money. Greater mood swings and depression.

Stage Five: Early dementia/moderate Alzheimer's. All symptoms are more pronounced now: more severe memory loss, including long-term memory loss, severe diminution in judgment and coordination; driving is a serious risk now.

Stage Six: Middle dementia/moderately severe Alzheimer's. Oblivious to current events, little or no long-term memory. Home care needed for dressing, eating, and toileting. Agitation and delusions are common, especially in the late afternoon or early evening ("sundowning"). Failure to recognize family members; suspicion of others. Wandering is quite common.

Stage Seven: Late or severe dementia. Speech becomes limited. Difficulty walking and sitting. Round-the-clock home care needed. End-stage immobility and unresponsiveness.

PART 6

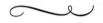

TIME TO SPEAK OUT

I'm not unhappy, just emotional. I'm happy to be alive and run around as I want, but I still want to be that other person, too— the person I was before. She's having a hard time.

I try not to make it anything big. I just want to get done what I'm supposed to do. It's not the worst thing. We still have romance in our marriage. Sometimes people are in the same house and never talk to each other. We're not like that. We have our moments, now, but we still love each other, and we still find things to laugh about together.

There's a joke we have.

"Hey," I say.

"Hey what?" Dan says.

"I forgot I had Alzheimer's."

The thing of it is, I do sometimes forget I have Alzheimer's because I feel normal, not because I've forgotten I have it. We can cook dinner together, watching the news on TV, and then sit down to eat, and Dan tells me what he's been up to, and I nod the way I always do. I may not remember everything he tells me, but I never did before I had Alzheimer's!

You know how it is in a marriage: sometimes you just listen to the sound of your husband's voice. And that's enough! Maybe *if you heard every word, you'd get bored! But you love him, and you love his voice, and it sort of washes over you like a favorite song. That's the way our dinners are now, not so different from how they once were.*

And I enjoy what I'm eating as much as I ever did. Well, maybe not if I messed up cooking it, which I sometimes do these days. I never did cook much from recipes, I just knew what a dish needed, sort of like a musician having an ear. Now sometimes I put in the wrong spice, or I forget I put it in before, and put it in again. You forget you put in the hot pepper flakes, and put them in again, you'll know it soon enough! But Dan usually cooks with me now, and keeps track of what I put in.

So the food is good—most of the time—and I don't have any trouble using a knife and fork, which is something Dan seems to keep an eye out for, which I find annoying. And then we usually go to the TV room and watch a movie. Doesn't all that seem normal, like just what everyone else does?

But then I get restless. I guess I have trouble following the movie if it's a complicated plot. I can't remember what came before. So I get up and go into my clothes closet to straighten my things. Or I take Bishop for a walk on the beach. I want to take that walk alone. I just need to be free for a while—on my own, not with Dan always standing over me. But he insists on coming, too, and so off we go, the three of us. If you saw us, coming the other way, maybe you had a dog, too, you'd think we were just a typical family, out for a walk with the dog. And in a way that's what we are.

TWENTY

New York City

Fall 2014

With Joan's help, we interviewed a wonderful home-care worker: a young Jamaican woman named Colleen whose last client had had Alzheimer's. Colleen had just become available, Joan told us excitedly; this was a stroke of good luck. I was reminded of that saying about doors: when one closes, another one opens. The reason Colleen was free was that her last client had died.

Colleen was well educated, well mannered, and imbued with a really positive attitude—impressive in her line of work. But I could sense B. holding back. After twenty-two years of marriage, I knew the first signals as well as the nose on my face. That very polite but slightly cool tone, the smile that departed just a little too soon, the tendency to listen and not ask questions . . . By the time she crosses her arms over her chest you know you're fighting for a lost cause.

Why? I wondered. But I knew the answer even as I posed the question in my mind. Colleen was a little too well educated, and maybe a little too attractive. The last thing B. wanted, in her diminished state, was a rival in her own house. Or so she felt. So excuses were made, and the post remained unfilled.

Meanwhile, I saw nothing wrong with putting B. alone on a jitney to Manhattan. A jitney, understand, is how most New Yorkers get to and from the Hamptons. Someone had the smart idea to call it the Hampton Jitney so people wouldn't think they were taking a bus. It *is* a bus, but a nice one, and parents feel fine about putting their ten-year-olds on it unaccompanied, as long as there's someone to meet them at the other end. I put B. on, told the driver to keep an eye on her, and said she'd be getting off at the first Manhattan stop, where her stepdaughter would be waiting for her. I needed to stay out in Sag Harbor and take care of business. Everything seemed under control.

The reason B. was headed in on her own was to buy a nice gown for a benefit lunch the next week. She still had all those gowns in her closet, but somehow none of those would do. I could have argued but . . . why? A new dress might lift her spirits, as it had before all this. In truth, I wasn't sorry to be getting a day to myself. Guilty—hell, yes. But not sorry. Anyway the lunch was a fund-raiser for a wonderful group called the Alzheimer's Drug Discovery Foundation. B. was to be the luncheon's honoree; she would be getting an award, and giving a speech, for becoming a spokesperson for Alzheimer's research.

The only problem with this plan was that Dana had gotten confused about when B.'s bus arrived in Manhattan. She'd thought it was due an hour or two later. When I called Dana to remind her the bus was arriving at 2 p.m., she exploded in that way I knew so well. "I'm on a bleeping train to Westchester to

see a litter of puppies. I thought she was getting in at three p.m."
Ever since Dana had given Bishop to us, she'd felt glum about
not having a dog of her own. The litter she was going to inspect
was of Italian mastiffs—Bishop's breed.

I called Ionia, B.'s friend and former stylist, who had volunteered to help B. do her gown shopping. Ionia had planned to
meet B. and Dana at Lord & Taylor. Instead, she rushed over to
Fortieth and Third to meet B.'s bus just in time. I would have
called B. to tell her Ionia would be greeting her, but I couldn't:
foolishly, I was still hoping we would find her lost phone, since
it had to be in the house somewhere. As a result, she had no
phone. Nor did she have any sort of identification necklace or
bracelet, let alone a GPS tracking device. Why, when being on
the jitney was as safe as being at home, a closed container from
point A to point B? Or so I thought.

Dana met them at Lord & Taylor, still steamed at getting the
times confused but grateful that Ionia was there. B., she knew,
would never go for a dress that Dana picked for her. It needed
Ionia's seal of approval.

Dana thought she would at least participate in the choice.
Otherwise, why be there? Instead, Ionia and B. emerged from
a dressing room with a purple dress in hand—purple being
the official color of the national campaign against Alzheimer's.
"This is the one," Ionia declared. Dana put it on her credit
card—B. no longer carried them with her, at my insistence; I
would of course reimburse my daughter. The dress was set aside
to be overnighted to Sag Harbor, and Ionia and Dana took B.
downstairs to find shoes for the dress.

B. hated the first four pairs of shoes Ionia showed her.

Worse, she was now confused. She couldn't recall what her new dress looked like.

The three of them went to take another look at the dress. "Okay, Mom, you got it?" Dana said. "This is the dress."

B. nodded, and the three of them trooped back down to the shoe floor. None of the next pairs met B.'s approval, either. Now she no longer recalled buying a dress at all.

"This is bullshit!" Dana exclaimed. Again they went to the dress floor; this time Dana took pictures of the dress. Now when they went down to shoes, B. could at least see what she was buying, and look for shoes that matched.

By the time Dana put B. on a 5 p.m. jitney back to Sag Harbor, both daughter and stepmother had calmed down. Dana always remembers—sooner than I do—that getting angry with B. is unfair and a waste of everyone's emotions. As for B., she just forgets why she was tense in the first place.

From Manhattan, the bus went straight to the Hamptons without a stop. Then it pulled into Southampton, and afterward came to Sag Harbor. I would be there when it pulled into Sag Harbor, right in front of the American Hotel.

Still, I couldn't help but feel guilty at the thought of B. alone on that bus, riding east in the dark. Would she know where she was, and why she was on it? Would she know I'd be waiting to meet her and get her safely home?

Or would she sit there wondering where she'd come from, and where she was going? And if she did, what would she feel then?

That night she got off right on time in Sag Harbor. I was there to greet her, and sweep her in to a festive dinner at the American Hotel. I remember thinking what a blessing it was that B. could still ride in and out of the city on the jitney herself. And that I'd been wrong to be so worried.

I wouldn't think that way for long.

A week later, we drove back in to the city together for the Alzheimer's benefit luncheon at which B. would be honored. We had written out a statement for her to read, and she was happy with it. For all that Alzheimer's had done to her, B. was perfectly capable of reading aloud a simple acceptance speech. Nor, I thought, would she have any jitters. Clouded as her mind was, B. was still the consummate professional. She knew how to work a crowd.

As the city skyline loomed, I snuck a sidelong look at her. She was fine. I was the one with jitters, I realized. Was I wrong to be doing this, putting her onstage in front of a crowd, even a sympathetic one? That's what Dana had felt. She would be there, too, but she wasn't happy about it. She felt the whole thing was a mistake.

As guests of honor, B. and I sat at a big round table in the Pierre hotel with family and friends. Along with Dana, there was Tichina Arnold of the television series *Everyone Hates Chris* and *Martin*. S. Epatha Merkerson, another television star, had played the lieutenant in *Law & Order* for seventeen years. Maurice DuBois, the WCBS anchorman, was there; so was Rashid Silvera, a longtime male model and dear friend of B. from her early days; Grayce Galioto, B.'s onetime assistant; Edward Robinson, B.'s oldest New York City friend; and Inez Richardson, head of the Metro-Manhattan branch of The Links, Incorporated, the national nonprofit group of African

American professional women. A lot of these friends hadn't seen or spoken to B. in weeks or months. Rapunzel hadn't let down her hair very often.

Paula Zahn, the glamorous television news anchor, was the luncheon's hostess, making her opening remarks to a packed banquet room of at least 250 people. Almost everyone there had some experience with Alzheimer's—a wife or husband, father or mother.

I thought B. was the only one who would actually have the disease, but I was wrong. Quite a few did, and came up to identify themselves that way to us.

B. sat beside me in the elegant purple gown she'd chosen, nodding and smiling as her old friends addressed her. She seemed more than fine: happy and animated. Only if you kept conversing with her would you realize something was wrong: a question repeated, a strange comment out of the blue. To one friend she said how lovely the luncheon was, so much so that she wished she'd thought to invite her parents.

There, too, was the renowned doctor who leads the Alzheimer's Drug Discovery Foundation (ADDF), Howard Fillit, along with a West Coast colleague and ADDF-funded researcher, Dr. Michael W. Weiner. As Paula Zahn explained in introducing them, the ADDF is totally focused on new drug trials. Leonard A. and Ronald S. Lauder, billionaire sons of the late cosmetics tycoon Estée Lauder, underwrite nearly all of the ADDF's administrative costs, so that all donations go straight to research. That leaves the doctors free to focus on the science, and work up clinical trials for the most promising new drugs.

Unfortunately, as Dr. Fillit told us, the news from the drug front wasn't good. The French drug company Sanofi had recently spent $1 billion on a new drug, to no avail. "To date, the pharmaceutical industry has spent well over ten billion dollars on drug research, including Phase 3 clinical trials that cost about three to four hundred million dollars each, and we have had a 99.6 percent failure. That can't go on forever," Dr. Fillit warned. Companies can't keep taking these huge risks without eventually saying this is too hard, and getting out. In fact, that is already happening. That is why we need philanthropy to create innovation and take risk, and partnerships between philanthropies, government, and industry to spread the risk."

There *was* one piece of good news: the PET imaging that now made possible clear diagnoses of Alzheimer's. At least, from now on, researchers would know that every patient in a new trial actually had the disease, rather than guessing from symptoms, only to learn after the three or five years of a trial that many of the participants had something else: another form of dementia, or just a naturally fading memory. "So instead of spending fifty million dollars on a trial with hundreds of participants to be sure we had enough with Alzheimer's, we can spend half that on a much smaller trial," explained Dr. Fillit's colleague Dr. Weiner. "Unfortunately, only 5 percent of Alzheimer's patients enroll in clinical trials. We need a lot more to join the fight." Dr. Weiner had an answer for that: a new, national sign-up operation he called the Brain Registry.

Now it was our turn. Paula told the crowd about B., and spoke of her courage. I guided B. to the microphone and gave her an encouraging squeeze. She started out fine—One-Take B. Then a wave of emotion washed over her, and she started to cry. Embarrassed, she turned her back to the crowd, and I stepped in to help. It was fine: no one in that audience was anything less than 100 percent understanding. I kept going until B. recovered and turned back to face the crowd. Then she threw her arms around me. "Don't I have a wonderful husband?" she called out. The crowd roared its approval.

The speech was put aside. For the next few moments, we just went on instinct and pure emotion, each of us speaking from our hearts. I don't remember all we said—it was a blur. But I do remember where it ended up. "Don't fear Alzheimer's," I said. "Hate it. And fight back—with the one weapon we have, money, to develop the drug that finally beats it."

We got a standing ovation. And I think I can speak for both of us in saying that for that moment, with all that love washing over us, we were really happy.

TWENTY-ONE

New York City

Fall 2014

Later that day, we stopped by our restaurant. How could we not? It's our baby. B. hadn't been there for two months and the staff was thrilled to see her. But they looked a little wrung out: it had been a challenging fall.

I felt bad for Dana, coming up to take over the place just as B.'s condition worsened. Not having B. at the restaurant every night was a blow to business—not one you could measure in dollars and cents, exactly, but in the loss of spirit, the flame snuffed out.

It hadn't taken Dana long to realize she had even bigger problems. We'd loved moving from B.'s first space on Eighth Avenue over to Theatre Row in 2000. *Theatre Row!* But the fact was, Theatre Row's glamour was fading. The old French restaurants on the block catered to an ever-creakier clientele. Joe Allen's still bustled, and Orso drew a tony post-theater crowd, but the neighborhood was changing, and not for the better. A lot of theatergoers bypassed it altogether for the cheap Asian/fusion restaurants and edgy new places in Hell's Kitchen to the west. As if all that weren't enough, a major new hotel was going up across the street. Construction stopped by the time we opened each night for dinner, but the site was an eyesore.

You could spin it different ways. Restaurants had their moments, and sometimes those moments passed. The Great Recession had hurt us bad, as it had the whole restaurant business. But even with the tough years that had followed, I'm confident we would have kept all three venues going—hung on until business bounced back—if not for B.'s condition.

Every night, as B. slept beside me, I lay in bed staring at the ceiling, thinking of ways to make it all work out. By 6 a.m. I was emailing and texting, working up ideas. But I could see the challenges ahead. B. Smith's *was* B.: the restaurants, the lifestyle books, the syndicated television show and radio shows, the four hundred products at Bed Bath & Beyond.

I did know now, from all I'd seen of how people related to B., that she was more than a brand: she stood for a way of life. Our mission statement, from back in the early 1990s when we'd started out, was "bringing people from all walks of life under one stylish umbrella." My goal now was to carry on the essence of who B. is, and what the brand stands for, in a time of racial division and animosity. We had a new mission statement, we agreed: *B. Smith is about bringing people together—period.* Not just for a restaurant meal or socializing at the bar. Bringing them together to help one another.

That felt like the right way to go—and doing this book would be a first big step in that direction. People from all over would rally around B. I knew how many people loved her; I had felt the power of that love. I wasn't just thinking about bed and bath products; I was thinking beyond. The humor of that hit me as I lay there, and I started cracking up. Bed Bath & . . . Beyond! No doubt the founders of the chain, in dreaming up that name, had meant it to refer to other rooms of the house. I was looking at it differently. "Beyond" to me meant getting the word out about Alzheimer's, getting people to rally around B., and coming together, black and white, Hispanic and Asian, to fight this disease together.

Meanwhile, I had a restaurant to keep alive, and one over-stressed daughter to help me do it. As much as I loved and admired Dana, I had more faith in getting to the big Beyond than I did in keeping B. Smith's on Restaurant Row from closing its doors after fourteen years. Privately, I thought we might squeak through the Christmas season, and shut down after that. We just weren't making enough to support it, and the losses were growing each month.

Fourteen years! It seemed like a moment ago.

TWENTY-TWO

NEW YORK CITY

1987–1992

Next door to the restaurant, all but unnoticed by hungry theatergoers, is a humble Lutheran church. That's where B. and I got married, nearly twenty-two years ago. So far, B. remembers that day as well as I do.

I first saw B. the way a lot of actors, directors, singers, and models saw her: holding court in the first bar that bore her name, on the scruffy side of Eighth Avenue at Forty-Seventh Street. I can remember the exact date: February 14, 1987. There was nothing scruffy about B. She lit up that room, a truly ethereal presence. B. Smith's was a hip bar in a fringe neighborhood, but I could see right away that B. herself wasn't hip. She was just this pure, gorgeous, gregarious woman who loved entertaining and had figured out a way to do it every night and make a living at it. More than that, she'd made a white-tableclothed restaurant for all New Yorkers, not just white New Yorkers.

On any given evening at B.'s place, you might see Richard Gere and Cindy Crawford, John F. Kennedy Jr., Steven Spielberg, Lena Horne, Harry Belafonte, Sidney Poitier, Denzel Washington, and more. B. Smith's had become one of the three or four places you went when the theaters let out. It was also a beacon of diversity in a town where black and white rarely mixed apart from the street and subway.

That first night I saw her, B. was wearing a fire-engine red bustier and red hostess gown—and managing to look demure while doing it. *Man,* I remember thinking, *it's like they poured chocolate into the perfect mold.* Unfortunately, I wasn't available to chat. I'd brought my wife, Jocelyn, to the joint for a Valentine's Day dinner and was about to bestow a pearl necklace on her. That's how I know the exact date I first saw B.

For the next three years, I came in as a friend, bringing expense-account groups whenever I could. I loved talking to B., but I never crossed that line. Later, B. would tell me how much she respected that. I was different; I didn't say corny things or act up like some of the guys.

I was a big, broad-shouldered guy coming up in the world of television ad sales and marketing, but no one had invited me in. I had just kept pushing until the first door opened. When you were a black kid from Bedford-Stuyvesant, that was all you could do. Push hard and talk fast. Or as the old saying had it, fake it till you make it. On my father's side, my family went back to 1754 in Virginia, the start of a long line of hucksters in the old-style definition of the word: they sold fruits and vegetables on steamboats, working their way up to New York. By the time my father came along, the riverboat life was long gone: he worked as a maintenance man. But he and my mother still had a bit of the huckster in them: they kept a numbers book. For a quarter or a dollar, your customers in the neighborhood bet on

different outcomes of the horse races that day: what numbers
the winning purses added up to, or what the last three numbers
of that total were. The keeper of the numbers book had to pay
out when one of his bettors won, but there was always enough
left over to make the business worth his while.

A teacher saved me, as teachers often do in a place like
Bed-Stuy. I got bused to an all-Jewish public school and nearly
dropped out: I could barely read. Mr. Vogelson saw some potential in me, and got me up to speed. For high school, I went
to the then all-boys Brooklyn Tech, an engineering school and
now one of the top schools in the city, and then Colgate University, where I dreamed of becoming a doctor. After graduating,
I found myself rooming with a guy who ran a job placement
firm. Just to help him, I'd go on job interviews when he didn't
yet have a qualified candidate. I'd get the job, and hold on to it
for four or five days until he could find a candidate who really
wanted it. I got offers right and left—I was the ideal African
American job prospect! Until I landed a job at Burlington Industries that paid so well I decided to take it myself. So I got
into the garment business, selling draperies to stores that no
longer exist, like Bamberger's and Abraham & Straus. That was
where I learned to kibitz. "Don't get mad," as one of my Jewish
friends liked to say. "Make a deal."

A chance introduction led me to a job selling ads for a radio
station in Memphis. Eventually I worked my way back to New
York, and to television, still as an ad salesman, but now for
Oprah, Jeopardy, and *Wheel of Fortune.*

Soon after taking my first wife to that Valentine's dinner, I
learned that B. had just published a book, *B. Smith's Entertaining and Cooking for Friends.* That made her the first-ever black

woman to come out with a tabletop entertaining and recipe book. I was awed, and proud for her, and strictly on a professional basis, I called a very influential friend on B.'s behalf. Marketing guy that I was, I could see exactly how to use this book as the basis for a whole new lifestyle brand.

The friend was Dick Robertson, head of Warner Bros. television distribution. His thing was syndication: coming up with new TV shows and selling them to stations around the country. I put a copy of B.'s book on his desk.

"There's a TV show here, Dick," I said. "I see it as one part cooking, but not a cooking show. One part lifestyle, but not a fashion and beauty show."

"So what the hell is it?"

"It's food, fashion, and fun, for a white and black audience."

"I still don't get it," Dick said. "What *is* it?" This is the way TV syndicators talk. At least, it's the way Dick talked. They hear pitches all day and they get pretty impatient with them. I could see I had one more play. "It's like Martha Stewart with rhythm," I tried.

Dick's eyes lit up.

"The black Martha Stewart," he exclaimed.

That was kind of crass but . . . yeah, I could roll with that.

The real Martha Stewart, as it happened, had just left Warner Bros. Dick wanted her back. First he spent $150,000 filming a pilot for B. Smith's show. Then he pitched it to Martha as a half-hour show to run before or after a half-hour show of her own. Yin and yang, sort of.

Martha hated it.

That was the end of our romance with Warner Bros.

Finally I worked my way in to see Irwin Gotlieb, president

and CEO of a hugely successful product marketing company called MediaVest. Gotlieb, unlike Robertson, was silent as I spoke, his hands clasped, very Zen-like. "Dan," he said when I'd finished, "we may have two clients for this." The clients were Procter & Gamble and General Foods. Success! They would underwrite the show, which was to say it would carry their commercials. It would be syndicated through Hearst Entertainment: sold to different local stations around the country.

The show made money—and history. Here was a black woman not talking about being black, just *being* black. A beautiful black woman with a stylish lifestyle that everyone, white and black, wanted to emulate. The show lasted for eight years. It led to two more entertaining books. It even hatched a magazine: B.'s own magazine, the first truly transcultural lifestyle magazine, with interracial couples, old-and-young partners, an Asian-themed Thanksgiving—you name it, we did it. By then, B. and I weren't just an item: we were married.

The romance began about three years after that first night I saw B. My marriage had ended when my wife walked out, leaving our young daughter, Dana, with me. I was struggling professionally, too. After a first successful year, a variety show I'd cooked up featuring singer Natalie Cole had been dropped. In retrospect, the show was a precursor of *American Idol.* But my sponsors had lost faith. Two weeks after that dopey decision, Natalie's new album, *Unforgettable,* came out and made her an international star.

I was drowning my sorrows in mimosas at another Eighth Avenue bar—not B.'s—when in she walked with a girlfriend, the two of them in natty double-breasted blazers. B. was wearing tight white pants with hers. "I need a hug," I said glumly.

Playing along, B. gave me one. "How do I get another of those?" I asked.

B. laughed. "Try using the phone."

A call led to a lunch date, at Caffe Cielo on what felt like our turf already: Eighth Avenue. We'd often chatted at B.'s bar, but a lunch date—that was a first. B. told me that her own first marriage, to an HBO executive named Don Anderson, had recently ended after three years. I fell in love with her right then and there. There's a light inside B., an honesty and kindness. You can see people who are beautiful but ugly inside, and then those who are not necessarily beautiful outside but beautiful inside. She had, still does, both types of beauty, inside and out.

I remember what she was wearing that day, too: a houndstooth jacket and an Annie Hall hat with a big brim pulled low so all you could see was her eyes and her smile. She kissed me on the cheek when I left her at the corner. I strode away, happy, hopeful, and then, after about ten steps, I thought to turn around. There, back at the corner, was B., still looking at me. I was special, she told me later; she was special, too. Soon we were inseparable, two sides of a coin. I called her Sweetie. She called me Big.

About eighteen months later—December 23, 1992, to be exact—we were married at the Lutheran church on Forty-Sixth Street: St. Luke's. We didn't yet have the restaurant space next to the church: we wouldn't open that B. Smith's until 2000. So after the church ceremony, B. and I led our guests in a parade up Eighth Avenue to the original B. Smith's on Forty-Seventh Street and packed the place until long after midnight.

Our wedding was written up in all its happy details in the "Vows" section of the *New York Times*. The article noted that

B. wore a ball gown the color of champagne roses and sparkly sequin-covered gloves. It went on to tell her story.

"Seven years ago, Barbara Smith, a model and an actress, opened B. Smith's Restaurant at West 47th Street and Eighth Avenue, next to a closed-down movie theater and across the street from a row of dilapidated tenements," the *Times*' Lois Smith Brady wrote. "Until Ms. Smith arrived the block was one of New York's bleakest.

"Some people now consider her corner a landmark," Brady went on. "As Edward J. Robinson, an interior designer and a regular customer at the restaurant, said, 'Anyone who comes in from out of town, I must take them to B. Smith's, then to the Statue of Liberty. There's always the possibility of seeing someone famous or in the news or in the know.' "

The article explained that we'd met at B.'s restaurant two years before—a slight chronological gloss. It noted that despite my day job in television marketing, I often spent evenings there now, doing everything from busing tables to coordinating the music. "I'm Barbara's cut man, and she's my cut man," I told the *Times*. "A cut man is the guy in the corner of the boxing ring who cleans up fighters and sends them back to battle. We'll always be in each other's corner."

Twenty-two years later, we still are.

LESSONS LEARNED

PICTURING THE PAST

I'm looking right now at a gorgeous picture of B. and me on our wedding day, B. in her cream-white dress with its lace-embroidered front, me in morning coat with my rose boutonniere, the two of us looking at B.'s ring under her sequined gloves. We look as happy as we felt that day, and every time B. sees that picture again, it cheers us both up. For all families struggling with Alzheimer's, there's a really helpful lesson in that.

The official therapeutic word for where I'm going here is *scrapbooking*. Family pictures are memory enhancers; an album of them is all the better. There's more than common sense in all this: not long ago I Googled my way to a list of twenty scientific papers on the subject, with catchy titles like "Therapeutic Implications of Portrait Photography in a Nursing Home," and "Photographs as a Tool in Memory Preservation for Patients with Alzheimer's Disease."

Once you get through their jargon, the studies make some sensible points. For the process of pulling a scrapbook together, they suggest enlisting the family member who has Alzheimer's. You know those piles of family pictures you always vowed to go through and put in albums? That time has come, with your loved one beside you. It's a great way to connect, to pass the time—and to create an enduring record of your loved one's life.

One bit of guidance is mostly to use larger pictures: easier to focus on. Start with a good-sized picture of your loved one smiling—the simple power of a smile to inspire a smile in return can never be overestimated. It puts your loved one in a good mood to thumb through the pages, and that's good, too.

Let your loved one's developing scrapbook become, as much as it can, a multigenerational story that works its way up through his or her life. Basically, a scrapbook is taking the place of your loved one's own repository of pictures—like a backup hard drive. You want to identify the faces in all the pictures; you also want to add recollections and key facts, writing them in beside those pictures. As with any scrapbook, other mementoes can be mixed in, too: diplomas, wedding certificates, a child's lock of hair, a military service medal.

Scrapbooking keeps the past fresh for the whole family, and helps children appreciate a grandparent who may have become sick before they knew him as he was. As the Alzheimer's progresses, it also becomes a means for a home-care worker to understand the soul inside the illness, creating more empathy and making for better care. When a severe-stage patient enters a nursing home or hospital, a scrapbook becomes that much more precious, giving doctors, nurses, and other patients some sense of your loved one's pre-Alzheimer's life.

For those who feel creatively challenged by the task of assembling a scrapbook—or for those just too tired to do it—a former nurse from upstate New York stands ready to do your family's scrapbook for you. Back in 2007, when her father-in-law got Alzheimer's, Brenda Siegfried made him a scrapbook in her own artistic style, with multicolored backgrounds and small objects like faux pearls attached to the pages. Family members would pick it up every time they visited, and turn its pages with him. "He could access it whenever he wanted," Brenda told me, "and it definitely helped his memory. He would talk about the people in the album, with a different story every time." Brenda did some online research on the subject that suggested scrapbooks might strengthen neural pathways and even create new ones. After her father-in-law's death, she started making scrapbooks for others, at minimal cost. That led to Scrapbooking Pathways, the business she basically started on her kitchen table.

"What I do is include just enough decoration to make it interesting but not so much as to overwhelm the person with Alzheimer's," Brenda explained. "Another scrapbooker may want to make it as beautiful as possible. Too much detail will distract the Alzheimer's client and it won't stimulate conversation." Brenda also does "reminiscence journals," in which she records family stories that can be told again and again.

When Brenda gets a new client, she conducts interviews like a reporter; gathers photographs, memories, and trinkets; and then assembles the book with that balance in mind. She offers two sizes of scrapbooks: 12 by 12 inches and 8½ by 11. Both contain twenty pages. Brenda says that each scrapbook takes her about twelve hours to complete. "I want to make it affordable," Brenda says. "My goal is to get an album into the hands of everyone who needs it, not to become a millionaire." (Her website is http://scrapbookingpathways.weebly.com.)

EMBRACING SOCIAL MEDIA

In our iPhone lives, I hardly need mention that taking pictures in an ongoing way can be both entertaining and helpful. B. and I take pictures of each other all the time, or put the iPhone camera on a timer and race back to pose for it. We have pictures of us with Bishop on the beach, walking along Main Street in Sag Harbor, eating lunch on the porch of the American Hotel.

Add those to the rooms full of photographs we have from B.'s earliest modeling days on through her entertaining books, the television show, and social meet-and-greet shots with everyone you can imagine, and we could assemble enough scrapbooks to create our own city-sized public library. Instead, we've made the sensible leap from scrapbook to Facebook.

Other social media would probably do just as well: Pinterest, for one, Instagram for another. But come on! We're in our sixties! It's all we've been able to do to manage one of these new Internet tools. Facebook gives us everything we need. As with scrapbooking, we post pictures of B. from earlier stages in her life, from our life together, and of us as a family with Dana. We'll add comments that come as often from B. as from me. I may have to tease them out of her, but I get them, and we post them. And then—my Lord, the responses! For better or worse, we don't just pussyfoot around in our postings. We tell it like it is. We talk about B.'s condition, the day's small victories or setbacks, and how we feel. I don't have the science to prove it, but I know that B. feels better for seeing new pictures on our Facebook page, and hearing the messages that come in. Old pictures may be even better. The other day I posted a poster of her from one of her early singing gigs. There she was, looking so young and glamorous, singing with Freddie "Rock Me Tonight (For Old Times Sake)" Jackson.

Like a lot of other Facebookers, I often post a picture of an especially tasty meal we've just whipped up. Once again, it gives Barbara a little lift—sometimes pulling her out of a funk. For a caregiver, that's no small thing.

Our favorite subject, though, is Bishop. "It's blowing 30 knots here," I posted in the midst of a real blizzard this winter, "a day not fit for man nor beast! But Bishop and I are beach bound!" B. never tires of the pictures of Bishop that we post on an almost daily basis. I can't quite describe what it is about his big, heavy head and those bulbous eyes, but that dog is *funny*. And B. laughs as much as I do just looking at him.

For me, Facebook has become a journal as much as a scrapbook—a place to vent frustration and, on a good day, to share some delight. "Just took the Bishop to the vet to get his nails clipped," I posted not long ago. "Walked home through Main Street, Sag Harbor, said good morning to at least 12–15 people. Walked home across the beach, no one was there, I just thanked God for the moment."

Post your own moments, your concerns, your dark and your light . . . it's one way to reach out to friends and share in the joy and the pain of this journey.

PART 7

WALKING IN HER SHOES

I don't feel different, but I know that I am. The slightest sad thought makes me cry. I never cried a lot before—not much in movies, not in real life, either. Now I cry if I hear annoyance in Dan's voice, or if he tells me I've had another sugary midnight snack I can't remember. Sometimes I cry when I'm alone, for no particular reason. They say crying makes you feel better. Not with me. It just makes me sad all over again.

That's not all I feel more sharply these days. I get angry at Dan—a lot. Usually it's something he says that I just flare up at. I never used to do that. I never had a temper. Now I do. The worst of it is: I don't remember, the next morning, why I was angry the night before. I see Dan wake up and give me a look, like: uh-oh, is she still on my case? And for the life of me, I can't remember what that case was.

Take that Alzheimer's luncheon. What do I remember of it? A big round table with my friends. Which made me feel really good, like they hadn't run away from me. I don't remember going up to speak, and I don't remember getting emotional, or Dan taking over from me, or me facing the crowd again and telling them what a wonderful husband Dan is. I mean—he is! I know that. But I don't remember that moment.

*I think maybe one reason I don't remember it is that it went
well. It seems like happy memories get blurred and forgotten now.
Maybe some little detail will be there. Like I remember talking to
a couple of people at that luncheon, but . . . that's all.*

*Ancient memories, many of them at least, are still unclear. The
other day I got to see my old friend Nancy Doll. Dan and I had
come into Manhattan, and Dan had business to do, so Nancy and I
got to spend the day together, just the two of us. I've known Nancy
since our early modeling days—she was a Wilhelmina model, too.
One year we went to Milan on our own and shared a room for
weeks at the Grand Hotel Milano. We'd go on shoots almost every day—sometimes together but usually separate jobs—and then
dance the night away. There were a lot of handsome rich Italians
giving parties at their villas in the hills, and to be honest, we got
invited everywhere. Nancy had a sort of hippie look: she liked to
wear her Frye boots, even to go out dancing. I wore heels and a
lot of clunky jewelry. That was one difference between us. But
neither of us gave those handsome Italians what they wanted. It
was a different time, an innocent time—for us, at least. We were
just having fun—so much fun.*

*That was what we talked about, the day we spent together:
Milan, and Paris, and Vienna, where I actually starred in a movie,
not that the movie ever got to the States. But for about six weeks I
was a movie star. It was great.*

*I know we talked about more recent stuff, but I can't remem-
ber much of what Nancy told me. I know she's back in Wisconsin,
where she grew up. I do know that.*

TWENTY-THREE

SAG HARBOR

Fall 2014

I think a lot these days about what it means when I tell B. that I love her. If I'm going to be honest—and there's no point in writing this book if I'm not—the love I feel for B. with Alzheimer's isn't the exact same love I felt for her on that wedding day twenty-two years ago, or even five years ago, before those first signs of difference seemed like anything more than the quirks of middle age.

B. is different. Life is different. My love is different, too. Yet what I've been thinking is that the love I feel for B. now is even deeper than the breathless excitement I felt when we first met. Passion for a beautiful, healthy partner is always a little narcissistic, you know? You feel that surge of happiness, your heart beats faster . . . those are the feelings in *your* chest, they're about how love makes *you* feel. I'm not even sure that's love. Maybe it's just infatuation. Or if it *is* love, the scientists tell us, then what we're feeling is pheromones—those biological exciters that buzz around our brains and bloodstreams, driving us to procreate and propagate the race. No matter how romantic you feel toward your lady love, pheromones last no more than eighteen months. That's science, man, not poetry. After that, the love calms down because the job is done, biologically speaking: you've done your bit for the species! Or you haven't, and those pheromones start swirling again as you encounter the next sexy vessel for your possible offspring.

Love for the woman you married becomes more about friendship and companionship than lust, and courtship is a memory in your rearview mirror, but that's fine. More than fine. Until one of you gets seriously sick.

You have a wife with Alzheimer's, and any last trace of frivolous romance goes away. What grows in its place is a new kind of love, a love that's *all* about her, not about you. It's about having her know you're there for her, doing whatever she needs. It's about caring for her, not abandoning her: to protect and to provide. I guess what they call that love is compassion. But that doesn't seem a big enough word for the feelings it stirs.

B., I should add, loves me in a way that's more profound, too. At least I think she does. She loves me as her husband, but also as her pillar of safety and support. She loves going with me and Bishop for a walk on the beach, sometimes talking, more often not; we have a new level of comfort with silence. She loves cooking with me, and curling up with me in bed to watch an old movie. Often, in one of those happy moments, she'll tell me how grateful she is for all I'm doing for her, and what I'll feel from her, when she does, is love of a kind as deep and devoted as mine for her.

Protect and provide—those are the watchwords for where we're at now.

TWENTY-FOUR

New York City

Fall 2014

A few weeks after that Alzheimer's luncheon, B. went into the city to see Dr. Howard Fillit, the founder and director of the Alzheimer's Drug Discovery Foundation, the nonprofit that the lunch had benefited.

We had known, even before the lunch, that Dr. Fillit was a leading force in the fight against Alzheimer's. Hearing him speak at the lunch made me realize that he was both a scientist and a physician, searching for promising drugs but also managing a small private practice, seeing Alzheimer's patients as part of his weekly schedule. From the way he spoke about them, it was clear that the clinical side was at least as important to him as medical research.

Howard had fought Alzheimer's for more than thirty-five years. Only in the last few years, though, had the fight become personal. He had watched Alzheimer's take over his father, step by all-too-predictable step. Howard's family had pleaded with him to take some extraordinary measure: as an expert in the field, weren't there strings he could pull, experimental drugs to try? He had none.

In his father's last days, hospitalized with Alzheimer's, Howard had sat with him, as helpless as any other son whose father was dying of the disease. As he stood up to leave, his father had had a rare moment of lucidity—like a rainbow. "I love you, son," his father had said. Howard knew that his father might not even remember his name. But the deep emotions of fatherhood had remained till the end.

At the luncheon, Howard had given me his card, put his cell phone number on it, and told me to call anytime. That had given me an idea.

Our doctors at Mount Sinai had done B.'s diagnosis and put her on various drugs; they had treated us with great sympathy and concern. But after the follow-up visit, we'd sort of drifted apart. We knew they were busy with new drug trials, and teaching, and seeing other patients. We had respect for all they were doing. We just needed someone who could answer a quick question when we had one. Howard, as we had come to know him, had told us to call whenever we wished. I'd asked him if he would agree to see B.; an office visit had been set up right away. This was a caregiver's lesson: never be shy about changing your doctor if your loved one isn't getting what you think she needs.

There was, I would soon see, another, quite horrifying lesson to be learned that day, but none of us—not even Howard—saw it coming.

That day, I put B. on the jitney from Sag Harbor to Manhattan. Dana would be waiting at the other end for her; she would take B. to Howard's office and then put her on the bus home. I wanted the day to clear out some of the piles of clothes and other stuff in the basement that B. was hoarding. The prospect of a day to myself cleaning the basement was looking pretty good. So was going that evening to the American Hotel for a drink or two, then having the jitney roll right up to the door. B. would get out, I'd be there to greet her, and we'd have a nice dinner before heading home for the night. Drinks and dinner at the hotel was one of the few pleasures from our former lives that we could still enjoy.

Dana was there at the New York end, right on schedule, to meet B. and walk her over to Howard's office on East Sixtieth Street. The day had turned chilly, and snow was predicted for the suburbs that night. There might even be snow for Thanksgiving, two days away. Perhaps to compensate, someone in Howard's clinic had cranked the heat up high: the waiting room was stifling.

Oblivious to the heat, Howard ushered B. and Dana into his office—an office as small and plain as Dr. Goldstein's at Mount Sinai. One thing you can say about Alzheimer's doctors: they aren't in it for the money. Or if they are, they're spending a lot of time in tiny offices waiting for it.

B. gave Howard one of her dazzling smiles and joshed with him as she took her seat. She looked fit and youthful, ready for a six-mile speed walk. Howard asked B. when she'd first noticed she had memory problems. "I don't really remember," she said, and described the facial tingling she'd felt all along. A few minutes later she described it again, exactly as she had before. And then a third time. Howard frowned. "Perseveration," he

said gently to Dana. "That's what that's called. And amnesia."
It wasn't good.

"Is she able to make phone calls?" Howard asked Dana
about B. "Can she dial the number?"

"If she wanted to make a phone call, she would, but she
doesn't," Dana said. "The remembering of the number might
be the hardest part, but also, she doesn't want to talk to
people."

"Well, I don't want to talk to everybody!" B. said with a
laugh.

"For her friends," Dana explained, "B. was the social person, the organizer. Now that she's not doing it . . . she's becoming socially isolated."

Also, we still hadn't found her phone.

"B., is there a reason why you don't want to do these things?"
Howard asked.

"It's hard to say," said B., and she started to cry.

When she'd recovered, Howard started probing for details of B.'s life at home—details that would give him a clear
sense of what stage of Alzheimer's she had entered. *Staging,*
they called it, which was diagnosing the neurological compo-
nents of cognitive losses, as identified by the loss of basic daily
functions.

"How is her speech, her language?"

"She has trouble with words and completing sentences,"
Dana replied.

"There's a name for that," said Howard. "Aphasia. Lack of
abstract thinking." Did B. still cook? he asked.

Dana nodded. "But her cooking isn't what it was. Of course,

when you cook at such a high level, as B. did—the level of a professional chef—you notice when things aren't quite as perfect as they once were."

"That, too, is aphasia. What household tasks does she still do?"

"She still does laundry," Dana said, "but it's not effective. If there are dirty rags on the floor, she'll wash those, but not the pile of clothes right beside them."

"Agnosia," Howard said quietly. "The failure to recognize what things are."

B. was not abusive, though, as many people with Alzheimer's can be. To Dana, and to me, it was just inconceivable that B. could ever be that.

"Sometimes she gets angry because she knows she's losing control," Dana said. "But she's such a happy-go-lucky person that even when she's angry I know she's not angry."

"Loss of emotional control, another executive function— very common," Howard said. "How about dressing? Can B. dress herself?"

Dana explained about the strange clothes choices—summer dresses with winter hats and shawls. But yes, B. could still put her clothes on herself. Still bathe herself, too, though if I didn't prod her, Dana felt, B. might forget to shower for days.

"The dressing problem is a good example of, among other things, apraxia," Howard explained. "The loss of the ability to sequence and conduct complex tasks. Ultimately, this leads to the inability to tie one's shoes, or even to feed oneself."

By now, Dana was hearing a pattern.

"Yes," Howard said, "the A's of Alzheimer's, they call it. Amnesia, agnosia, aphasia, apraxia, apathy, and loss of executive function or abstract thinking."

Howard wanted to know if B. still drove.

"Dan doesn't like it when I drive anymore," B. chimed in, "but I'm not afraid to drive."

"She should not be driving at all," Howard said sternly. "There are problems with reflexes and judgment at this stage."

"She walks into town now," Dana assured Howard.

That brought up another concern: identification. "Do you have a bracelet that says who you are and explains you have Alzheimer's?" Howard asked.

B. did not.

"I'm worried she might get lost," Howard said. "What kind of identification does she have?"

"We cannot find her purse," Dana said with a sigh. "I'm looking for the gold one and the black one. She has not had her cell phone for a couple of weeks, either."

Howard frowned. "She must have an identification bracelet that says she has Alzheimer's," he said. A cell phone was critical, a handbag with pieces of identification, too. But as the last weeks had shown, they could be lost. That's why the bracelet was even more important.

A bracelet, no driving—and no alcohol. In an already impaired brain, alcohol could push things over the edge.

B. nodded meekly as Howard ticked them off.

"Has she lost weight?"

"Not that much," Dana said. It was true: I'd kept off the weight I'd lost on our Mediterranean diet, but B. had gained some back by eating sweets.

"How about her appetite?"

"Horrible!" Dana said. "She eats all these sugary snacks at night."

"Dan has the cookies!" B. exclaimed with a laugh. "He won't even share the cookies with me!"

It was true: I was the cookie monster, keeping them out of her reach.

Howard laughed with her, but then turned serious. "I want B. to eat whatever she likes," he told Dana. "The worst thing is if she loses too much weight. I'm not so concerned about preventing a heart attack in twenty years because she has too much cholesterol. At this point it's about *not* losing weight. I don't care if she has sundaes every day."

"You'll have to convince Dan," B. said.

"I'll write you a prescription for cookies," Howard said with a grin, and proceeded to do just that. Just to be sure, Dana photographed it with her iPhone and forwarded it to me in Sag Harbor.

Along with eating regularly and well, even with a few prescribed treats, the best thing B. could do at this stage, Howard said, was exercise daily. He was pleased to hear that we had gotten a trainer for B., and that he was working with her three times a week. It wasn't enough, but it was a start. "Exercise releases factors from the muscles that help the brain," Howard explained. "Don't just exercise three days. If you possibly can, exercise *every* day."

Howard looked through the thin new file he had for B. so far. "I see you have a living will and a health-care proxy," he said approvingly.

"I don't want to hear that," Dana said.

"It's good, though," Howard said. "It expresses her wishes."

As yet, the file didn't have B.'s blood tests and brain scans from Mount Sinai. If Howard was going to be her regular doctor, he would need them. "Please request the records from Mount Sinai," he told Dana. "They're your property." That was good to know.

Howard paused.

"I want to talk about home care," he said, looking hard at B. "Dan says he is stressed-out—and beyond. You and he both need home care—right away. I would like to start with at least four hours a day, probably five days a week—at the minimum."

I had explained, when I first met Howard, how the conversation went whenever I brought up home care with B.: how she said yes, "as long as it's someone we like," and then ruled out every prospect she met. Howard said he understood completely: taking on home-care help signaled a loss of privacy and independence that no one wanted. But that, Howard said in so many words, had to change.

"B. is no longer mild stage," Howard told Dana, using the three-stage model. "More like middle stage, based on how long she's been sick, as well as on her cognitive and functional disabilities. We need to start putting the long-term care plan together that keeps B. safe and lets Dan have some time off. It's not just about where we are now but where we're going to be in six to twelve months from now."

To confirm his gut sense of what stage B. was in, Howard put her through a few cognitive tests. He showed her a page with circled letters and numbers, and drew a line from A to 1, then from B to 2. "Can you continue the pattern?" he asked B.

She could not.

"I'm going to say some words I want you to remember," Howard said. "Face, velvet, church, daisy, red."

B. could recall only the first two. Howard repeated them to her and asked her to keep them in mind as they did other tests.

"Tell me words that start with the letter *F*."

"Finger . . . food . . ." Those were the only ones B. could suggest.

"Can you tell me the names of ten animals?"

A long pause. "Bunny . . . chicken . . . a horse, a cow . . ." and then a longer pause. "I'm glad Dan isn't here!" B. said with a laugh.

"I'm not," Howard said soberly. "I wish Dan *was* here to see this."

Each of the tests probed one or more brain functions. The A-1, B-2 test? Reasoning, or as doctors put it, executive function and language. Animal naming? Executive function and memory loss. "What do shirts and shoes have in common?" Howard asked B. "They're both covering something and making something easier in your life, as far as the shoes go." Abstract reasoning.

Finally Howard asked B. to recall the five words he'd told her to keep in mind. She couldn't remember a single one.

"Was one of the words a color?"

"I don't know."

"Was it yellow?"

"Maybe."

"Was it a flower?"

"I don't remember."

"What is today's date?" Howard asked.

"I don't know."

"What year were you born?"

"I'm not sure," B. said. "Ninety forty-nine, maybe, or 1942."

B. didn't know what year it was. She didn't know what city she was in.

"B. is much further along than we thought," Howard told Dana. "Her social personality is very strong and maintained, but it's a veneer behind which there is much less than appears—or than I thought."

The parts of the brain that handled these functions were being devastated, one by one: the temporal lobe (memory and learning), the amygdala (tying emotions to memories), the frontal lobe for executive function (judgment, reasoning, planning, working memory, and emotional control). Alzheimer's was like Sherman's army, leveling everything in its path, the disease spreading in a now well-established pattern.

Until now, Howard had maintained a doctor's demeanor: cordial and concerned but a bit detached. It seemed to fall away as he turned back to B. "Here's the thing," he told her gently. "I want you to be happy, and that's what we're going to do for you—keep you safe and happy. That's the only thing that's really important. I want you to have a schedule, so that you have fun and are safe every day. As far as medicines go there may be a couple of others I want to prescribe but I need to have your chart sent over from Mount Sinai. Above all, I need you to accept someone in the house now—a home-care worker who can help you with all these things. Will you do that for me?"

B. nodded. "Yes," she said softly, "I will."

And then the office visit ended, and the worst eighteen hours of our lives as a family began.

TWENTY-FIVE

NEW YORK CITY

November 25, 2014

From Howard's office, Dana walked B. to the nearest jitney pickup: Lexington Avenue near Fifty-Ninth Street. The sky was the dirty white of possible snow, darkening on this late November afternoon as the bus drew up. Dana helped B. find a seat, then told the driver her mother had Alzheimer's. Could the driver keep an eye on her, and be sure she got off not in Southampton—the first stop in the Hamptons—but in Sag Harbor, the stop after that, where I would be waiting for her? The driver said he would—or so Dana recalled.

Three hours later, as the bus rolled up to the American Hotel, I was there to greet it. One by one the passengers disembarked. I was sure that B. would be the next one, or the one after that. She wasn't. Panic gripped me as the last passenger climbed down. I bolted up the bus steps to ask the driver what the hell had happened. No, he said, no woman fitting B.'s description had gotten off in Southampton. "Well then where is she?" The driver just shrugged and said he had no idea. Even if he'd seen her get off in Southampton, he told me defensively, he couldn't have stopped her. He couldn't stop someone from getting off the bus. Well then, why had he said he would?

At that Southampton stop, there's an inside waiting area where you can sometimes get coffee and a bagel, or even a glass of wine. Surely B. had gotten off in Southampton and was waiting for me there. Where else could she be? A jitney employee checked: no luck. The waiting area was empty.

Now the full impact of this hit me. B. had vanished. She had no phone. She'd lost the gold handbag in which she kept her driver's license and credit cards. I'd put some secondary identification in a little clutch bag she'd taken with her. But how likely was she to have it still with her? She could easily have left it on the bus.

Here's the stone-cold truth: you can never truly, fully appreciate how much you love your partner until you feel you might have just lost her forever. The woman I'd married—the woman I'd loved since that first night I saw her on Valentine's Day, 1987—was already gone, her mind diminished, her very character wearing away. Yet she was still my B., still the woman I could hold, still the sweet companion who told me how grateful she was that I took such good care of her. I wasn't feeling like I was doing such a good job taking care of her now. My B. had just vanished, with little or no awareness of wherever she was.

I called the police but learned it was too soon for them to conduct a search. As the evening hours passed, and a cold rain came on, all I could think of was whether she was safe, and where she might be, and how irresponsible I'd been in letting her get on that jitney alone. The phone kept ringing, but it was never her, nor anyone calling to say they'd just run into her. I talked to Dana a dozen times, and got an earful each time: my daughter reminded me in no uncertain terms that she had disapproved of my putting B. on the jitney before, on the trip to get her fancy gown. Why had I gone ahead and done it again? It was stupid, and thoughtless, and now look what had happened. Under her recriminations, I felt Dana's own guilt, as strong as my own. I knew she felt that by putting B. on the jitney, even at my urging, she was to blame as well.

After a sleepless night, I had to face the reality that something awful might have happened to her, and that it was time for the police to get involved. The Southampton jitney stop wasn't in Southampton village; it was on busy County 39, a four-lane road lined with car dealerships and medical buildings all closed by 8 p.m. There was no nearby diner or coffee shop where B. might have huddled through the cold and rainy night. I'd checked those farther away—no luck. Any decent person who had come in contact with her would have called the authorities by now. To me that left only two possibilities. Either she'd walked into the woods alone and spent the night outside, or some psychopath had abducted her.

Alarmed now, the police put out an Amber Alert for B. throughout Suffolk County. They started filing a more formal missing person's report, too.

At a friend's suggestion, I called the local television news station and the local radio station. Then I took it a step further: I called the major New York City newspapers. I had mixed feelings about that; it was like swinging a bat at a beehive. But as mortified as B. would have felt if she'd been able to understand it, I just felt it was another way to get the word out—a card we

could play because B. was well-known. Why not? I'd do anything to get her back.

By 10 a.m. that Wednesday, a media caravan had descended
on our Sag Harbor house. There were video cameras and mi-
crophones and lots of people—for me it was all kind of a blur.
Fox News and CBS News were the first to get out the word;
USA Today soon followed. "An alert has gone out for famed restaurateur and former model Barbara Smith, known as B. Smith,
who has Alzheimer's and has been reported missing on Long Island. . . . Police in Sag Harbor, where she lives, confirmed that
there is an open, active missing person investigation seeking
Smith, and asked for the public's help in finding her."

I'll never forget that Wednesday morning, how slowly the
minutes passed. The press stayed encamped at the house, waiting, as I was, for news. Emails and calls were coming in con-
stantly, from all over the country and abroad. Apparently those
first news stories online had gone viral. I'd known a lot of people out there loved B. I had no idea how many. All those voices
of love and concern—it was incredible. I wished I could have
appreciated them more. All I could think about was B. I kept
looking out at the rain, cold and raw, hoping she wasn't exposed
to it, hoping wherever she was she was safe, and warm, and dry.

And then, as shockingly as it had begun, the ordeal ended.
Out of the blue at about 2 p.m. that day came a call from a Sag
Harbor friend of ours, Terry Steiner. Terry and her husband,
Roger, had a house in Sag Harbor, but that's not where Terry was.

She was in Manhattan.

Terry had run into B. at a diner called La Parisienne on Sev-
enth Avenue between Fifty-Seventh and Fifty-Eighth streets.

Terry had just happened to walk in, and seen B. sitting at one of the tiny tables. B. greeted her warmly, but looked disheveled and disoriented—and wet.

Terry hadn't heard that B. was missing, but she did know B. had Alzheimer's. Still, she might have said hello and moved on. After all, B. was just a block from our old apartment on Central Park South. Clearly she'd gone there because it was familiar to her; La Parisienne was a favorite quick-bite place for us. And despite her appearance, B. was cheerful as always. But Terry was sensible enough to take action—and for that, I'll always be profoundly grateful to her. Not having my cell number, she called our restaurant on Forty-Sixth Street; a restaurant employee then called Dana, and Dana called me.

Dana was a stew of emotion, grateful and relieved but also frustrated. First she had lost her birth mother; for the last seventeen hours, she had had to fear that the stepmother she loved as her real mother was gone, too. I got it—and felt awful. No more jitney rides alone for B., that was for sure.

Terry stayed until Dana arrived to take B. to her Chelsea apartment. B. was, of course, happy to see Dana, but in the way she might have been to see her after a little trip to the store. She was *thrilled* to see the newest family member in Dana's tiny studio apartment: Sansa, the Italian mastiff puppy Dana had just gotten to replace Bishop, named after a character on the HBO series *Game of Thrones*.

After Dana's relentless questioning, the mystery was solved. B. hadn't gotten off the jitney in Southampton and then boarded a bus back to New York, as I had imagined. She'd never gotten to the Hamptons at all. Between Fifty-Ninth Street, where she got on, and Fortieth Street, the jitney's last stop before leaving Manhattan, B. had forgotten why she was on the bus—and gotten off at Fortieth Street.

The details were in bits and pieces, like shards of a broken mirror. B. had walked the streets of the city all night—that much was clear. She was wearing heels, and her feet were badly blistered. Apparently she had walked first up to Harlem—she said as much—then all the way down to Battery Park. At some point she had taken a ferry to Staten Island; she remembered someone recognizing her, and singing songs with a group of people. She'd come back on the ferry, and then resumed walking, all the way up to La Parisienne. Whether she'd huddled for some hours in a doorway like a homeless person, or possibly come by the restaurant on Forty-Sixth Street long after it had closed for the night, and tried to get in—these were details we'd probably never know. They were lost already in B.'s fog.

As soon as I could gently ease the media and various concerned neighbors out of the Sag Harbor house, I drove in to Manhattan to Dana's apartment. Dana was relieved, and B. was happily playing with the puppy: as Dana had said to Dr. Howard Fillit, B. was more and more like a puppy herself. She apologized for scaring us both; she knew enough to know she'd done that. How much more she knew was hard to gauge.

At least I had B. back, and she had us. For all we had lost, we were still a family, and on the day before Thanksgiving, that was a lot to be grateful for. Dizzy with relief and happiness, I put B. in the car and drove her out to Sag Harbor as I should have done the day before. The next week, she would have no recollection of that ride.

With all the excitement, it somehow didn't occur to me to

ask if B. was hungry until we rolled into Sag Harbor. She was. What did she want? Not kale, or berries or sardines—none of that Mediterranean diet tonight. "Hot dogs," said B. with a grin. "That's what I want."

So we went to the market and bought a dozen Hebrew National hot dogs, along with Häagen-Dazs Dulce de Leche ice cream and various kinds of Pepperidge Farm cookies. Back at the house, we ate and ate, happy as fridge-raiding kids. Then I helped B. into a hot bath, put her into warm, dry pajamas, and we got into bed to watch an old movie with our ice cream and cookies.

The next day was Thanksgiving. No turkey dinner for us: we were just thrilled to sleep late and spend the day together.

I was exhausted, but thoughts were churning in my mind. For me, as B.'s caregiver, this was a wake-up call I'd finally heard. Joan, our strong-willed advisor from the Alzheimer's Disease Resource Center, had warned us before: no more leaving B. on her own. I'd thought the jitney was an exception, and Dana had certainly made it clear to the driver that B. had Alzheimer's and mustn't be let off before Sag Harbor. How had he heard that message at Fifty-Ninth and Lexington, and forgotten it by Forty-Second Street?

At the end of the day, though, I was still the one to blame. However inattentive the driver might have been, I was the one who'd made the choice to put B. on that bus in the first place. I made that choice in the State of Denial, a place I intended never to visit again. A lot would have to change—right now. Yes, we would get home-care help, hopefully someone B. liked, right away, but if not, then someone she *grew* to like. Saying no to one candidate after another was no longer an option. We would get

B. an Alzheimer's bracelet and a GPS tracking device. We would not let her ride on the jitney alone; we would not leave her home alone without someone to watch her. All this, plus daily exercise and that healthy diet, we would resolve to do. We would also have to face the realities of medical insurance. How much would all this cost, starting with the daily home care? Would Medicare pay for it, now that B. was sixty-five? If not all, how much?

But I wasn't just thinking about us. I wanted to know why medical science hadn't gotten further with this disease. Why had no one yet come up with a treatment or cure? We'd gone public to help eradicate the stigma of Alzheimer's, especially in the black community, and I wanted us to do a lot more. I wanted to do more than the occasional TV appearance and newspaper story. I wanted to use our platform to say to the scientists and doctors, the drug companies and policy makers of America: let's do something *big* about this. More than thirty years ago, AIDS had swept out of Africa like a global storm, and many had died, but then activists had pushed drug companies, and policy makers and politicians had helped, and out of that devastation had come a "cocktail" of drugs that turned AIDS from a killer into a manageable disease.

Where was our cocktail? Where was our Manhattan Project for Alzheimer's? Where was our Hail Mary pass for the 5.2 million Americans suffering with Alzheimer's right now?

To be smart about that, to know what the hell I was talking about, I wanted to learn what was going on—in the labs, at the drug companies, in the halls of Congress. I wanted to know— and then I wanted to help push it all where it needed to go.

LESSONS LEARNED

Cognitive Tests, Games, and Books

Dr. Fillit conducted quite a number of cognitive tests with B. and brought, of course, a lifetime of medical expertise to analyzing the results. The fact is, though, that anyone with a fading memory can download cognitive tests and be his own judge of whether the results justify voicing concern to a primary care doctor. And for loved ones in the first, mildest stage of Alzheimer's, a number of brain exercise tests and games may just help slow the progression of the disease. Even if the science is sketchy on just how much they help, they sure can't hurt.

The Alzheimer's Association lists a dozen or so memory game and test sites. Some are free, some aren't, but none are expensive. Among the free ones: www.fitbrains.com, www.aarp.org/fun/puzzles, and www.setgame.com. The fee sites include http://mybrainteasers.com, www.happy-neuron.com, and www.brainhq.com.

Our personal favorite is www.lumosity.com. It's a trip! You can try it for free at first, and it's well worth the time. Before you know it, you're looking at cards, trying to remember if the new card matches the card you just saw—or steering different-colored trains into their proper train sheds, clicking to turn the tracks that get them where they're supposed to go. You tailor a program of games to your needs: memory, attention, speed, flexibility, and problem solving. And then you do the games several times a week. It's like push-ups for the brain—but more fun—for about fifteen dollars a month.

Here, too, are just some of the books that also have puzzles and games to test and strengthen the brain:

Get Your Brain in the Fast Lane, by Michel Noir and
    Bernard Croisile
365 Exercises for the Mind, by Pierre Berloquin
The Memory Bible: An Innovative Strategy for Keeping Your
    Brain Young, by Gary Small

And finally, two books for Alzheimer's patients no longer able to play games quite as challenging:

The Best Friends' Book of Alzheimer's Activities, by Virginia
    Bell, David Troxel, Tonya M. Cox, and Robin Hamon
Alzheimer's Activities That Stimulate the Mind, by Emilia
    Bazan-Salazar

WANDERING

Wandering is an all-but-inevitable symptom of Alzheimer's, a direct consequence of damage to the brain. The wanderer may have intended to go from point A to point B but gotten lost en route. She may feel determined to get oriented on her own—like a subway rider who emerges from a station confused, for a moment, about which direction to head. Only the wanderer, unlike the commuter, can't get her bearings. That may make her anxious, and further impair her ability to find her way home. She may just wander out of curiosity or boredom.

One good measure is to have an ID bracelet or necklace made for your loved one with name, phone number, and nature of the disease ("Alzheimer's" or "memory impaired"). A new generation of GPS-equipped locator devices has made a huge impact on the issue. Some are worn on the wrist, others are pagers, still others are attached to cars. A loved one's family can follow a wanderer's path on-screen, as satellite signals track her. The Alzheimer's Association offers Comfort Zone, which also has a 24/7 hotline with a national search program. (See Resources for more details.)

Wandering is exacerbated if the patient moves to a new home, or starts going to a new daily care center; she may be unable to process that this is where she should go.

Wandering confused in Manhattan is, by definition, potentially dangerous—but in a rural area, in perhaps very cold weather, it can be life-threatening. Most wanderers go no farther than a few miles from their homes, and can generally be found by police. Maddeningly, when asked, they tend to deny they're lost. That was the case with B. Even after wandering all night and morning, she still didn't tell our friend Terry that she was lost. Terry had to sense that herself.

Along with providing the loved one with a GPS tracking device, helpful measures include hiding the car keys, not leaving a wanderer in the car alone, and providing as much of a daily schedule for her as possible.

For the caregiver, wandering can seem a form of rejection. It isn't. It's just part of this dreadful disease.

The A's of Alzheimer's

There's some debate in the field about how many "A's" of Alzheimer's there are: four, five, or more. I count eight. Here they are, in alphabetical order:

- Agitation: nervousness and alarm, with a tendency to restless movement
- Agnosia: a difficulty with processing sensory information, leading to the inability to recognize familiar objects, tastes, sounds, and other sensations
- Amnesia: loss of memory
- Anomia: inability to remember names
- Anxiety: persistent and excessive worry or concern
- Apathy: general indifference, inability to feel optimistic and happy
- Aphasia: inability to express oneself through speech
- Apraxia: the loss of fine motor skills

PART 8

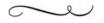

STALKING AN
UNSTOPPABLE
DISEASE

I don't remember the doctor's visit, or Dana putting me on the jitney. I don't remember why I got off and started wandering. I do remember it was the evening, so it didn't seem . . . out of place. And I remember I felt good. I wasn't scared or worried. I felt free! I was taking care of myself, having an adventure. I know that's not a really good thing now, I know everyone was horrified and thought I was dead. I didn't mean for everyone to worry! But sometimes you just need to be on your own.

My only problem was my heels. They were red, and pretty high. If I'd known better, I wouldn't have had those heels on, because they were killing me by the end of the night.

I remember I went up to Harlem. There wasn't anyone in particular I wanted to find. I was just wandering, seeing what I wanted to see—because normally when you're with other people you have to see what they want to see. I knew to be watchful of who was looking at me or who was following me on the streets, because who knows what someone might be? But nothing happened to worry me at all.

Then I headed down to that boat—the Staten Island Ferry. Maybe the Staten Island Ferry isn't the best thing in the world, but *it's still a boat, and it looked beautiful at night, and it was going somewhere—that was enough for me.*

So I walked down to the ferry, and got on, and I started talking to people, and they started talking to me. It was like at the restaurant; it seemed natural to me. I think someone recognized me. "Hey, that's B. Smith!" They started telling me where they were from, it was like a party on that boat, looking over the water. And then I remember we were singing—all of us, together. Teenagers, and at least one older person. I can't remember the songs but I know we were singing. It was cold, but I wasn't shivering. I wasn't smart enough to shiver!

I didn't get off on the Staten Island side. I stayed on and rode back to Manhattan, and then I walked back up to Midtown. I knew there was something missing—our apartment! I knew it wasn't ours anymore. But it felt right to walk up to our old neighborhood, and I guess that's how I ended up in that diner. It felt familiar. I don't remember who started talking to me there. I do remember Dana's puppy when I saw it at her apartment. It was so beautiful.

I don't remember Dan driving me out to Sag Harbor, but I know he told me how everyone had been looking for me. Not in a bad way. It hadn't bothered me, but I know it wasn't a good thing to go wandering like that—I won't be going away like that anymore.

When I came back to Sag Harbor we went to the American Hotel, and everyone was so nice. It was like being at home with the family—it's pretty much like that down there. Everyone was so nice.

TWENTY-SIX

SAG HARBOR

Fall 2014

Within two days, B. and I were interviewing more home-care prospects. I could sense B. still holding back on hiring anyone to come into our home. She tells other people she knows she needs help, but when the doors close and it's just us again, I get, "No, no, no, I don't want some kindergarten student getting in my way."

How do you force your wife to accept home-care help when she doesn't want it? I'm telling you: it's not as easy as just hiring the person and bringing her into your home. I knew that unless B. accepted her, we'd all go through hell. With B., the best way was to coax her, bit by bit, until she came around. As awful as the last week was, I still thought we had time to ease B. into the home-care idea.

This wouldn't be easy, not in any sense. Even on a limited basis, Colleen or whomever else we hired would cost at least $1,000 a week. So $52,000 a year—just for starters. A lot more for round-the-clock help—which was in our future, I knew. In all, maybe $100,000 a year before long. We had resources. But I could see how easily Alzheimer's drains an average American family's savings.

As the horror of that night began to recede, I started thinking about how to plan financially for this future, while also doing good and making a difference. Two ideas popped into my mind. I wanted to keep B.'s successful line of home products on the shelves and selling, as they had for fifteen years now. But I also wanted to introduce a new line of all-natural white goods—sheets and towels and such—that we would call B. Smith Basics. These would have no chemicals—100 percent natural. This tied in with our whole campaign of a healthier diet, and healthier living through keeping it simple. Keeping healthy was, so far, the best advice that doctors had for keeping Alzheimer's at bay. I hadn't decided whether those products would include messaging about Alzheimer's, but they might. Maybe part of their proceeds would be donated to research. I wanted Bed Bath & Beyond to help us raise global awareness and money for Alzheimer's. Maybe this could do it. I had another idea about how to do that: with a stamp.

A stamp for Alzheimer's awareness, with B. Smith as the face on the stamp.

This wasn't so crazy as it seemed. Not long before, a breast cancer awareness stamp had raised $80 million for breast cancer research. A surtax was added to the price of a forty-nine-cent stamp—five cents, I think it was. The forty-nine cents went to the federal government as usual; the surtax went to the good cause. The catchphrase just came to me: "If you want to make a difference, put a stamp on it." And why not bring Bed Bath & Beyond into the picture? They had a mailing list with 37 million customers. If I could get them to use B. Smith stamps on their mailers, that could be serious money for Alzheimer's research. I started making calls to educate myself on what all this might involve.

Already I knew one very deserving recipient: the Alzheimer's Drug Discovery Foundation (ADDF), founded and run by our new doctor, Howard Fillit.

Howard was the one I wanted to see now. He was the key. I wanted all his advice on dealing with B., from ID bracelets to home care. But I wanted to talk to him, too, in his other capacity, as a leader in the fight against Alzheimer's. I wanted to know what was happening on the front lines of drug research—and I wanted to raise buckets of money with B. Smith Alzheimer's stamps to help him find the right drugs that much sooner.

Howard's ADDF offices are on West Fifty-Seventh Street. He has a staff but really, the ADDF *is* Howard. He's the one who was persuaded by Ronald and Leonard Lauder, sons of Estée, to start a major philanthropic effort back in the late 1990s to accelerate the discovery of new drugs for Alzheimer's.

Up until that point, as Howard explained, scientists were scattered around the country studying the genes that might or might not cause the disease. We had doctors holding clinical trials for drugs that might or might not make a difference. We had big drug companies paying for some of those studies, and the federal government paying for others. And still we had no drug that actually treated or cured the disease—partly because more research was needed, and more money to fund it, partly because all those efforts were separate and apart from one another: silos on the Alzheimer's landscape. A private foundation could cut through some of the red tape. It could choose the most promising drugs and pay for Phase I and Phase II trials. It could finance new biotechs and spin them off to big drug companies if the data looked good. The Lauders knew that Alzheimer's research was one long trail of failures. But *something* had to be out there, and private philanthropy was maybe the best hope of finding success.

In his ADDF office, Howard gave me a short history of Alzheimer's.

In 1906, a German psychiatrist named Alois Alzheimer told colleagues of a curious case of dementia in one of his female patients, aged fifty-two. The patient had had memory loss, hallucinations, and fits of jealous rage at her husband. After her death, Alzheimer put her brain tissue under a microscope. Utilizing some dyes to stain the tissue, he noted abnormal deposits in the brain that he called "senile plaques." Dr. Alzheimer also saw "dense bundles of fibrils" that he called neurofibrillary tangles. The tangles appeared to be in dying neurons. Later, scientists would determine that the tangles were primarily made of a protein they called tau. Dr. Alzheimer's role in making that link between amyloid and the tau-related dementia it seemed to cause in a relatively young woman—a form of presenile dementia— led colleagues to name it in his honor. There it remained, all but ignored, for the next sixty or seventy years.

The problem was that most people, including neurologists, saw senility in older people as part of the normal aging process. You got to your seventies or eighties, things happened. Maybe your memory loss was a lot worse than the next guy's, but so what? Your time was about up.

In the late 1960s, some pathologists in London did autopsies on people who died with "senility" and found the same pathology that Alzheimer had described in 1906. It was then that senility went from being thought of as a normal part of aging to being recognized as a disease of old age. In the early 1980s, a researcher named George Glenner took the next step, isolating the senile plaques from human brain autopsy tissue and determining that a major component was a protein called beta-amyloid. Scientists thought they had found the "cause" of Alzheimer's disease.

This was also the time that the whole science of genomics emerged. Suddenly scientists were sequencing the DNA of animals and, eventually, humans, seeing a whole new world of genes and the proteins they coded—proteins that gave you curly hair or blue eyes or a prominent nose. Some of those proteins appeared to have flaws or mutations; those flaws seemed to cause diseases. The DNA for beta-amyloid was sequenced. Mutations in the DNA coding for beta-amyloid were found in people with "early onset" or presenile Alzheimer's, like the first patient described by Dr. Alzheimer. For a while the whole scientific community thought for sure that a breakthrough was around the bend. All they needed was a molecule that blocked the flaw from causing the disease. But the next two decades passed, and no easy answer appeared.

Maybe Alzheimer's was caused by a more complex process. Maybe nothing the scientists had assumed was what they thought. Maybe not even amyloid plaques were involved. True, they appeared in Alzheimer's patients. But maybe they didn't cause the disease. Maybe they were just a result of it.

The plaques, after all, can be present in individuals who never develop symptoms of Alzheimer's. Howard, for one, remains a skeptic about amyloid. There are many forms of amyloid, he says, found in various parts of the body, and often they are not the cause of a disease but the product of it. He thinks amyloid was just the obvious culprit—the low-lying fruit, as he puts it. In the end, he feels amyloid plaques could prove a neurological decoy. Despite many billions of dollars spent on clinical trials attempting to prevent or remove the beta-amyloid, none of these drugs have worked in humans until very recently, and far larger trials—both for safety and efficacy—are needed. Meanwhile, he calls for funding other strategies and trying other targets.

To Howard, and others, the likelier suspects are the so-called tau tangles, the actual dying neurons. Maybe amyloid plaques simply enable the tangles to form, and the tangles are what kill the cells. Or maybe the plaques and tangles have nothing to do with each other; maybe the tangles form on their own in order to do their killing work. Maybe protecting the neurons is the best way to prevent Alzheimer's.

Back in the mid-1980s, both sides—those scientists arguing that amyloid plaques caused Alzheimer's, and those pushing the tau tangle theory—expected genomics to settle the debate in a year, maybe two. But the standoff persisted, as some of the early excitement over genomics subsided. With its amazing DNA sequencers, genomics could zero in on genetic flaws associated with a disease, but it couldn't say whether those flaws actually cause the disease—only that they're associated with it. Big difference. The cascade of new drugs expected to come of genomics has proved to be more of a trickle, as trials reveal adverse effects, or the drugs simply fail to work.

"The challenge of finding a drug is more daunting than ever," Howard told me. "It's harder than putting a man on the moon." The universe of molecules that *could* be drugs is almost infinite. Yet so far, we have just ten thousand on the market for the whole kit and caboodle of human disease. That sounds like a lot—but it's a lot smaller than infinity. And only about five hundred of those are unique drugs; the rest are combinations of the original five hundred, and new ways to administer them.

Finding that next drug is so hard that 90 percent of researchers at pharmaceutical companies spend their whole careers working on drugs that never get to market. Either the drug doesn't perform as hoped or it has some harmful effect. Getting a molecule to do what you want it to do—every time—and not cause any harm in the process, is really, really hard. And maybe with Alzheimer's, as Howard explained, no single drug will do the trick. "Look at AIDS," he said. "It turned out we needed a whole cocktail of drugs for that."

Meanwhile, costs continue to climb. A recent study out of Tufts University has shown that getting a new drug through all three phases of FDA government-monitored trials and out to market now costs $2 billion. Baked into that figure, as Howard had pointed out at the ADDF luncheon, is the cost of failure: the cost of the last drug or two that a company invested in to no avail and hopes to get its money back on. It adds those losses to the cost of the new drug, hoping to recoup them in the end.

Facing those odds, the drug companies have become risk-averse, to say the least. Howard sympathizes with them; he thinks drug companies, despite their bad rap, are almost heroic for taking the risk with billions of dollars to test new drugs again and again. But he also feels the breakthrough drugs for Alzheimer's will come from cutting-edge biotechs and university labs doing clinical, early-stage research. They're the kind of efforts the ADDF is backing. They're where innovation will happen. Now it's only a question of backing the right one.

TWENTY-SEVEN

NEW YORK CITY

Fall 2014

In the sixteen years that ADDF has been in operation, Dr. Howard Fillit has steered over $70 million from the Lauders and others to fund more than 450 programs in eighteen countries, including more than 65 biotechs. Some are start-ups that would have gone unfunded without the ADDF, since venture capitalists in the medical field are wary of small biotechs in general, and Alzheimer's in particular.

The biggest triumph so far for ADDF has been funding the original research that led to PET imaging for the brain—the same technology that showed those plaques in B.'s brain and confirmed her diagnosis. The story of neurological PET imaging also shows how the ADDF works—and how it may yet find the ultimate Alzheimer's drug. In 2004, it began funding a start-up program at the University of Pennsylvania that had the idea of injecting a radioactive molecule that could bind to the beta-amyloid in the brain and track it as it went through the brain. The places where the radioactive material bound to the amyloid indicated amyloid plaques. In 2005, the idea was spun out as a biotech called Avid Radiopharmaceuticals, with some $7–8 million from investors to ramp it up. Five years later, the giant drug company Eli Lilly bought Avid for almost $800 million. In 2012, the PET amyloid imaging test from Avid became the first diagnostic test for Alzheimer's to market with FDA approval.

Imagine! One could detect the presence of beta-amyloid in the brain without having to do a brain biopsy or an autopsy! This would surely improve the diagnosis of Alzheimer's disease, showing with certainty who had it—and who didn't. That was big, but as Howard is the first to admit, PET brain imaging doesn't treat the disease, let alone cure it. Medicare, as a result, refuses to pay for the test—because the test doesn't change the outcome. Everyone still dies.

Howard is furious about that. Before PET imaging, as he points out, diagnosing Alzheimer's was a guessing game based on symptoms. Here was a test that clearly distinguished who had Alzheimer's from who didn't. And for people with memory problems, the reassurance that they don't have Alzheimer's, but might have a treatable cause, could be priceless. Wasn't that worth perhaps three thousand dollars of reimbursement per patient? Certainly, there are many other tests for other diseases that cost as much or more. But not according to Medicare. So today, only those who can afford the test get it.

Despite that impediment, PET amyloid brain imaging has been a breakthrough in how brain researchers do clinical trials. Today, practically all patients who enter into a clinical trial for Alzheimer's receive the test. It turns out that about 30 percent of people entering these trials prior didn't even have the disease. This really confounded the studies, making them very difficult to interpret, and could account for some of the drug failures. PET imaging has eliminated that problem.

The test has also led to game-changing prevention studies. Now, as Howard told me, we can see Alzheimer's developing up to twenty years before someone begins to exhibit the first symptoms. This is truly revolutionary and suggests a future in which early detection leads to early-stage drugs that make a real difference at last.

I took all this in, but finally I held up my hand. Okay, I said, I got it. Alzheimer's was a challenge, genomics hadn't given us the magic bullet, and PET imaging, as helpful as it is, doesn't cure or stop the disease. But surely there were drugs in the pipeline—somewhere—that an insider like Howard knew about, right? For an awful disease that afflicts 5.2 million Americans? Above all I wanted news of drugs on the way for early-onset Alzheimer's, the kind that B. has. I knew that genes played a key role in early-onset; why not new, gene-targeted drugs? I didn't know much more than that, because I'd shrugged off the scientific jargon; I'd assumed it was all over my head. Now I wanted to know it all, and found I could take in a lot more than I'd thought. When your loved one is fighting a deadly disease, it's amazing how much you can retain, after all, of the genetics, the neurobiology—all that stuff. Because maybe if you learn it, and concentrate on it more intensely than your busy doctor, who has so many other patients to tend, you might hit on something that could, perhaps, be useful. Some treatment not yet tried, some alternative medicine not yet in common use. I mean, why not, right?

Howard explained that we do know more about the role one particular gene plays in early-onset Alzheimer's. It's called APOE, and all of us inherit a form of it from each of our parents. The question, with each parent, is *which* form we inherit. APOE-e2 and APOE-e3 are good guys: they move cholesterol and other fats through the bloodstream and out through the liver. In fact, people with APOE-e2 are protected from Alzheimer's disease. Without APOE-e2 and APOE-e3, those fats would just accumulate, restricting blood flow and leading to heart disease, ultimately to heart failure. But then there's APOE-e4, which is definitely a bad actor. Because it contains a genetic flaw, it gums up the job that APOE-e2 and APOE-e3 do, and clearly has something to do with Alzheimer's. If one of your parents passed on the APOE-e4 variant to you, your chances of getting early-onset Alzheimer's go up. If you have double APOE-e4—one from each parent—your risk of getting Alzheimer's is 15 to 20 times that of the normal population. Also, you'll get the disease a decade sooner, so sixty-five rather than seventy-five years old, on average. That doesn't mean everyone with APOE-e4 will get Alzheimer's—many will not, which unfortunately only increases the mystery of how APOE-e4 works.

Scientists have known about APOE-e4 for over twenty years—but that doesn't mean they have a drug for it yet. They don't. "The genomics is scientifically interesting," Howard said, "but translating a gene into a drug is incredibly hard."

Also, the fact that APOE-e4 is involved doesn't mean that APOE-e4 is the *cause* of Alzheimer's. It may just be a risk factor. All scientists know for sure is that it's *associated* with Alzheimer's and seems to increase the risk that more plaques will form and the cascading effects of Alzheimer's will follow.

How to block APOE-e4 is the question. Two of Howard's funded research teams are developing a gene therapy using APOE-e2 to counteract APOE-e4. The idea is to isolate the DNA that codes for APOE-e2 (the "good" APOE), put it into a very safe virus—like putting a passenger into a little space pod—and then inject it into the brain of a person with APOE-e4. The APOE-e2 may offset the bad effects of APOE-e4. That may lessen the odds that amyloid plaques will form and that a person will get early-onset Alzheimer's. But does that mean a drug is on its way for early-onset patients like B. who've already gotten the disease and are passing into its middle stages? No, Howard told me, it doesn't.

With late-onset Alzheimer's, coming up with new drugs may be even more of a challenge because it involves aging. APOE-e4 is associated with it. But so are various other aging-related processes and symptoms. We know the cast of characters, most of them anyway. But we don't know nearly enough about how the play unfolds. "The only thing we know is that aging is the leading risk factor," Howard told me.

That isn't to say that aging causes Alzheimer's. There isn't necessarily any direct cause-and-effect link between the two, or else everyone would get Alzheimer's as they age. But something in the biology of aging is clearly involved.

"When you've been on earth for seventy-five or eighty years, getting repeatedly hit by toxins, inflammations, and free radicals, not to mention actually hitting your head—think of soccer players or football players or boxers—you've probably sustained neuronal injury," Howard explained. "One of the ways the body may respond is by producing amyloid. And it appears the clearance mechanisms for amyloid in the brain work better

for young people, less well in older people. But there are many
other mechanisms to cause neuronal injury as well."

We can't help having been knocked on the head now and
again. Nor can we help having lived sixty or seventy years with
all the neurological wear and tear involved. So many of us may
accumulate our share of amyloid plaques by the time we reach
old age. But just having amyloid plaques doesn't mean you get
late-onset Alzheimer's, either. Some octogenarians have lots of
plaques and never forget a phone number, much less get the
disease. Amyloid does seem to play a supporting role. Maybe
even a lead role. But not, perhaps, the only role. So what else is
involved? Mostly, what those other triggers have to do with is,
in the broadest sense, lifestyle.

Just in the past few years, Howard explained, the science
has become much clearer on the subject of health and its con-
sequences, for better and worse, on what they call the noncommunicable diseases: heart disease, diabetes, hypertension, and,
yes, Alzheimer's. Fitness and a good diet keep them at bay; lack
of exercise and a couch-potato diet help bring them on. The unmistakable sign of the latter is obesity, so rampant in America
in every age and socioeconomic category. Obesity, and the bad
habits associated with it, has been shown to be a risk factor for
Alzheimer's.

Diet and exercise aren't just beneficial in some vague, feel-
good way, Howard explained. They literally turn on genes that
help us. A whole new science called epigenomics regards genes
as a sort of circuit board, to some extent under our control.
Simply by changing our diet, we can cause a whole circuit board
of genes to be either active (or "expressed") or inactive ("not
expressed"). How cool is that? More and more, the interaction

between genes and the environment we expose them to is being seen as hugely significant. Unfortunately, these diet and exercise genes are probably most effective in fighting Alzheimer's early on—ideally, years before the disease can be diagnosed, when mere wisps of Alzheimer's-like symptoms go unnoticed.

Exercise and diet, Howard told me, actually stop the brain from shrinking. "With cognitive aging, our brains shrink by about point-four percent a year," he said. "Recent studies have shown that with brisk daily walks over a period of months, certain parts of people's brains actually get bigger.

"The brain is like a muscle," Howard added. "The more you build it, the more you will protect it from all the toxicities that affect it."

Okay, I said. Exercise, diet—I got it.

And no drinking, Howard added. That went for caregivers, too, not just patients.

The recent findings about Alzheimer's and lifestyle haven't led to new drugs yet, Howard said. But there *is* some good news in all this. Drugs that work for the other noncommunicable, lifestyle-linked diseases—hypertension, diabetes, heart disease—might work for Alzheimer's, too. *Repurposing*—that's what they're doing with these established drugs now.

The great advantage of repurposed drugs is that they're approved and on the market for at least one condition already. So that $1–2 billion in development? It's already been spent. And proving that a drug designed for some other disease also happens to work against Alzheimer's is a whole lot easier and cheaper than starting from scratch. Repurposing drugs isn't like getting secondhand stuff. Some repurposed drugs have gone on to make far more money by their new use than their original one. Exhibit A: Viagra, originally designed for pulmonary hypertension.

So far, unfortunately, Viagra appears to have no effect on Alzheimer's. But other hypertension drugs may. One class focuses on angiotensin receptors in the blood that under the wrong circumstances can narrow blood vessels, increase blood pressure, and force the heart to work harder. Angiotensin receptor blockers (ARBs) can help relax the blood and reverse that process. It turns out that in the part of the brain called the hippocampus, where Alzheimer's begins, there are also angiotensin receptors that are neuro-protective. The ARBs may be able to improve brain blood flow and decrease the deposits of amyloid that grow into amyloid plaques in animals. A recent study at Johns Hopkins University showed that certain blood pressure medicines—in the same bailiwick as hypertension drugs—led to a dramatically lowered risk of Alzheimer's, as much as by 50 percent. But as with so many of these promising results, this one needs a lot more research.

A diabetes drug called liraglutide looks promising, too. It helps diabetics take up insulin. Turns out, it does good things for the brain, too. Specifically, it seems to prevent the buildup of amyloid plaques in animals, to repair neurons, and to keep synapses working. The brain, as a result, works better and can better cope with stress and toxic influences. One study with mice suffering from late-stage Alzheimer's found that liraglutide managed to reduce amyloid plaques in the brain by 30 percent after two months. A first clinical trial of liraglutide, funded by the ADDF among others, is under way.

For heart disease, of course, statins such as Lipitor are used to lower the cholesterol that blocks arteries and leads to trouble.

In recent years, statins have seemed to hold the promise of protecting against Alzheimer's, too—so much so that they've gone through three clinical trials for it. Unfortunately, they failed to meet their clinical test goals. But Howard is still cautiously optimistic about statins. "We don't know if statins failed because they don't really play a role—or because we treated people too late," Howard explains. But at least one new study—not a clinical trial—suggests that in high doses, statins help prevent dementia. So here again, the jury is out.

Another repurposing possibility is drugs for rheumatoid arthritis. Enbrel is a so-called biologic drug that has proved effective in blocking the inflammation of psoriasis as well as rheumatoid arthritis; it seems promising as an agent to fight inflammation in the brain, too. That could make it a critical tool against Alzheimer's, since inflammation is an important part of neuronal injury. In a recent test, Enbrel slowed cognitive decline in only a small subset of Alzheimer's patients, so more clinical studies need to be done.

The Mediterranean diet, by the way, is also an anti-inflammatory and antioxidant diet. There's no doubt that inflammation, designed to help us heal, can also do us harm. That happens when our immune systems, for complex and not wholly understood reasons, start attacking us instead of defending us. That prompts the reaction of inflammation—sometimes directed at our nervous system, sometimes at our skin, and in the case of Alzheimer's, our brains. The foods we eat can cause, or prevent, oxidation and inflammation. In addition to the staples of a Mediterranean diet—the fruits and vegetables, the fish, the olive oil, and so forth—certain spices, and garlic, can also fight inflammation. Dr. Christopher Cannon of Harvard Medical School treads a careful line here. "Although specific studies haven't yet been done on some of the popular anti-inflammatory eating plans, the related Mediterranean diet has been studied and is associated with improved outcomes in some diseases."

The Mediterranean diet isn't the only prospect that nature gives us. All of us have a protein in our brains called brain-derived neurotrophic factor, or BDNF, and nerve growth factor (NGF), which do really good things for us—and may do even more than we know. Both BDNF and NGF affect the function of the hippocampus, that part of the brain so integral to memory. When we're young, they help brain cells grow and communicate with one another, literally increasing the brain's size and capabilities. Throughout our lives, they keep doing that; the process is what's called neuroplasticity. At the same time, BDNF and NGF may protect our brain cells from injury related to inflammation or oxidation, or even from the toxic effects of beta-amyloid.

The only problem with BDNF and NGF is that they're hard to use as drugs. They degrade in the stomach if taken orally, and would be hard to administer by injection. Howard's foundation has funded scientists at Stanford and elsewhere to develop drugs that mimic the effects of BDNF and NGF and protect against all the various kinds of brain injury that natural BDNF and NGF address. The drug developed at Stanford that mimics NGF is now in clinical trials. Meanwhile, we can all try to boost our BDNF, not only with the right diet and exercise, but with omega-3 oils. Though the science on omega-3s indeed remains uncertain, there's no harm in them and—anecdotally at least— much potential benefit. Yet another possible BDNF booster is sunlight. A team at Leiden University in the Netherlands has found that blood levels of BDNF increased among their participants in the sunniest months, and decreased during those short Scandinavian winter days. Maybe heading south for the winter makes even more sense than we knew.

Vaccines are another promising approach. Monoclonal antibodies, a kind of vaccine against beta-amyloid and even against tau, are in development by a number of pharmaceutical companies. So far, the drugs have not been very promising, though in a recent small clinical trial, an anti-beta-amyloid vaccine from Biogen raised hopes. Eli Lilly has an anti-amyloid antibody, too. Neither so far does the trick completely, the way we expect vaccines to do. Still, both vaccines slow cognitive decline in early-stage patients. So vaccines do have potential; but it's likely we will need a cocktail of drugs, as in AIDS, to come to grips with the disease.

If he had to guess, I asked Howard, where would he say the first significant Alzheimer's drug will come from? Which approach? And by when?

Howard shook his head.

"We don't know where the first effective drugs are going to come from." On his desk, he keeps a little plaque his daughter gave him. "It's a quote from Einstein," he said with a wry smile. " 'If we knew what we were doing, we wouldn't call it research.' "

Damn that disease. I'm no scientist; no politician, either. I can't invent a new drug, nor a cure. But I can see how desperately one is needed, and maybe in my own way I can help raise awareness—help put pressure on our public and private sectors to steer more money to research and get the job done.

By now I've realized that the chances of a silver-bullet drug coming along in time to save B. are slim at best. I've had to confront that reality after all these months of seeing her get steadily worse. Her all-night wander broke my heart—made her even more precious. It's also forced me to accept that we aren't at "mild stage" now. Just keeping B. happy in the time she has left—that's what I'm aiming for now. But for all the others who come after her—beautiful people with dwindling minds—I can push, and pressure, and politicize, until we get the breakthrough after all.

TWENTY-EIGHT

NEW YORK CITY

Fall 2014

So that was the report from the pipeline. No silver bullet, but maybe some repurposed drugs by 2020, likely for early-stage patients: the goal for managing—not curing—Alzheimer's. For a geriatrician like Howard, the drug story is hopeful but frustrating. The story in home care is downright maddening. Drug research and home care: those are the two sides of the Alzheimer's crisis. The real tragedy is how much better home care could be handled right now, without any new miracle drug.

B.'s disappearance, it turns out, is an all-too-typical outcome of insufficient, unsupervised home care. I blame myself—clearly I shouldn't have let B. get on that jitney—but she'd done it before, put on at one end by Dana with me at the other to meet her, and nothing had happened. How were we to know, without some guidance, at what point she could no longer do that? "Most medical practice is about writing a prescription," Howard explained. "But this illness requires care management, and attention to home care, and advance planning—and prevention. What happened to B. is a perfect example of how bad care leads to bad outcomes, and it has nothing to do with pills."

With Alzheimer's, the patient usually sets off a first cascade of bad outcomes herself. So scary is the disease that most people simply ignore their worsening symptoms of memory loss—for years—and don't go to a doctor for them. When they do, they usually go to a primary care physician. They mention memory loss—names, dates, that kind of thing.

That's when the system—our troubled medical system—impacts care. The average office visit for a patient with a primary care physician is about eight minutes. Our current structure of medical insurance, including and especially Medicare, the national insurance for 97 percent of elderly people, creates precisely the wrong incentives through its in-office reimbursements. A doctor who spends an initial hour assessing and diagnosing Alzheimer's, and then another hour with a patient and his or her caregiver for essential Alzheimer's counseling, will soon find he can't pay the rent.

As we knew now, the pills available, like Aricept, at best have a modest, stimulating effect on a patient's memory. They do nothing to halt the progress of the disease, much less reverse it. A doctor will likely prescribe one of those; he may also prescribe an antidepressant for some patients, as B.'s doctors did for her, and that, of course, can make a patient feel better—while her Alzheimer's is getting worse.

Thanks to the system, what happens to the patient after that initial visit is . . . not much. The patient goes home, takes her pills, and copes, as does her caregiver—until a crisis such as a hospitalization becomes unavoidable. Most patients aren't even "staged," or properly and fully assessed, which is to say they aren't given the various cognitive and functional questions that Howard gave B., as a new patient, to determine at what stage of the disease she is, and what her capabilities and home-care needs are. Those visits take time: B.'s initial visit at Howard's office lasted roughly an hour, far too long for the system. "This is what a geriatrician does," Howard explained. "Unfortunately, there are very few of us out there."

Staging and overall assessment can help with a whole range of options, both for the patient and her caregiver. Howard gets passionate on the subject. "To the primary care physician I say: your role with Alzheimer's, as with any chronic disease of old age, is not just to prescribe medicine but to care for the patient. There are so many caregiving needs! Can she drive, use the phone, manage her finances, plan a bus trip to get food? And later: can she bathe, dress herself, groom herself, feed herself, walk?"

A primary care physician should counsel his patient—and the patient's caregiver—on all these needs, and be in regular touch about how they're being met. But that's hard, if not impossible, with the current system. Most doctors can't take that time. They also lack the training. Fortunately, there are a growing number of "memory centers," often based in neurology practices generally at larger medical centers, that are offering comprehensive diagnostic services and multidisciplinary care for Alzheimer's. In France, the government has set these up all over the country.

"A large part has to do with multidisciplinary care—that's what's required," Howard told me. "A knowledge of aging is important; knowing how to deal with the medical and nursing and social work and other issues that arise from Alzheimer's and require community services, up through the end-stage issues like malnutrition and incontinence and pressure sores, and even palliative and hospice care. The average doctor doesn't—and really can't—do this. Geriatricians, and some of the memory centers, do sometimes have the staff for this, but they're few and far between in the US." Recently, Medicare tried to address this problem by providing a reimbursement for doctors and their staff to provide "chronic care management" for patients, including home-care guidance to patients and their caregivers. Sounds great, right? Certainly a step in the right direction, but the reimbursement is about forty dollars per patient per month and requires documentation. The average doctor's office overhead consumes about 50 percent of his salary, so we're talking twenty bucks, take home, before taxes.

For the caregiver and his loved one, home-care needs translate into one word in red neon letters: MONEY. And until the system changes, there's no avoiding that.

The costs begin long before a caregiver throws in the towel and hires home-care help. They come in terms of lost wages—first for the patient, then for the caregiver. Often a caregiver is forced to quit his or her job altogether. That loss may have larger ramifications. Imagine a hospital nurse who has to leave her job to care for her own mother at home. That's the hospital's loss, too.

Not many Americans can afford the $100,000 average yearly cost of home care. For those over sixty-five, Medicare steps in, which means we all pay. Only Medicare doesn't pay all the bills—or even what it purports to cover. Certainly long-term care is not paid for by Medicare, and generally not adequately by Medicaid. Alzheimer's is often "under-coded" by health-care providers in clinical practice and hospitals. That means some medical needs aren't deemed important, and so aren't covered. Other costs are reimbursed, but only partly. All too often, a family's resources get whittled down to the point that they have to go on Medicaid: they are, in fact, destitute. Alzheimer's has wiped them out.

By now I could see there was not just one war to be fought, but two. Pushing to get funding for new drug trials was one. Coming to terms with the long-term, human tragedy of Alzheimer's was the other. And who suffers the most disproportionate losses in both wars? That, too, was clear to me now: African Americans, the same ones who'd suffered the most in every major US conflict from the Civil War on.

I needed to know more about that.

LESSONS LEARNED

The Inevitable Question of Insurance

I've learned that fighting medical insurance companies for coverage of Alzheimer's-related expenses can be as nasty and unrelenting a struggle as taking on the disease itself. Here are the realities:

B. was sixty-four when I took her to the doctor who tried the depression patches on her back. She was still sixty-four when she got those cognitive tests, from which that doctor concluded she probably had Alzheimer's and prescribed a PET imaging test. So B. didn't have Medicare yet, but we did have Empire Blue Cross Blue Shield. I had thought those visits would be covered. No such luck. Both doctors were "out of network."

Unfortunately, the PET imaging wasn't covered, either. So that month, when the bills came, I had a bill for $1,000 or so from the depression-patch doctor, $4,000 for the cognitive tests, and another $4,000 for the PET imaging. Oh—and our monthly premium bill from Empire Blue Cross Blue Shield for about $1,000. What had we gotten from Big Blue? Absolutely nothing.

If there was any blessing on the insurance side, it was in B.'s birth date: on August 24, 2014, she turned sixty-five, and I found myself filling out her Medicare forms. Now that she's covered, the costs are far lower than they would have been pre-Medicare. Far lower. But that's not saying Medicare is a free lunch. It covers office visits, but only after a deductible of about $400 in our case, as a family subscriber. It doesn't cover PET imaging, either.

Medicare covers inpatient hospital care with most of the doctors' fees included. Medicare Part D also pays for most—but not all—prescription drugs. Over the disease's long progression, other needs are covered less completely, if at all. Medicare will pay up to one hundred days a year of skilled nursing home care under limited circumstances—and only after a hospitalization! It's not clear what family caregivers are supposed to do the remaining 265 days of the year with loved ones who have moderate to severe Alzheimer's and need daily help, and who don't want or need to be hospitalized due to their condition.

Long-term nursing home care is not covered by Medicare—period. If you don't have the money to pay for a nursing facility, you just turn your home into a nursing facility—it's free!

For patients judged to be near the end of life, Medicare will pay for hospice care done in the home, or in a nursing facility, or an inpatient hospice facility.

Okay, a nice sendoff, at least.

Just out of curiosity, I called Empire Blue Cross Blue Shield to ask what they would have covered if B. had stayed on their rolls. In other words, if B. had gotten early-onset Alzheimer's at, say, fifty years old, and had only private insurance to see her through the duration, what would that have meant? I reached a nice benefits lady named Catherine, who kept having to check on the details but always came back on the line with them. Catherine's father had died of Alzheimer's, as it turned out.

Catherine confirmed that office visits are covered, after your deductible, whatever the deductible is in your plan. She said that some tests are covered, too, once you get a specialist's referral. But that's only if the specialists are in network. I already knew that my own doctors were out of network. Just one of those catch-22s.

I learned that Empire does cover home-care visits by a skilled nurse, but only up to forty visits a year. The nurses, of course, have to be "in network." That could mean someone who lives nearby, but more likely much farther away. The fee? A deductible first has to be met. Then Empire pays 95 percent of the "allowed amount."

What is the "allowed amount"? I asked.

Catherine told me it's the amount negotiated for a patient's care between his doctor and his insurance company. As Howard confirmed, there isn't much, if any, negotiating to be done by the doctor: Empire calls the tune. So if a test costs $1,000, the insurance company may decide that its allowed amount for that test is $200, and pay 95 percent of that. The doctor either accepts that deal—or declines to accept Empire Blue Cross/ Blue Shield.

And so it went with hospital and hospice care: always that reassuring 95 percent that Empire Blue Cross Blue Shield would pay . . . but always 95 percent of the "allowed amount" between Empire and a doctor, which in most cases was so low that the doctor might end up refusing to perform that service for the "allowed amount."

OTHER ALTERNATIVE TREATMENT HOPES

In addition to BDNF, a number of other alternative therapies offer hope for Alzheimer's, but none are proven, as yet, and some may actually be detrimental to your health. Here's a roundup:

Acupuncture

Some studies have indicated that acupuncture can address the depression and insomnia often associated with Alzheimer's.

Aromatherapy

The idea that essential oils, derived from plants, can have soothing effects is generally accepted. Whether it goes so far as to improve cognitive skills in patients with Alzheimer's is unproven, though possible. The Alzheimer's Society specifically notes lemon balm (*Melissa officinalis*) and lavender oil as possibly helpful with Alzheimer's, though again, the proof isn't there as yet.

Bright Light Therapy

The common symptom of "sundowning," which B. may have experienced as extra anxiety and restlessness on that Very Bad Night as the winter sun set, may be offset in the home by special bright lights. In bright light therapy, as the Alzheimer's Society explains, "a person sits in front of a light box that provides about 30 times more light than the average office light, for a set amount of time each day. One small but well-conducted study showed promising effects of bright light therapy on restlessness and disturbed sleep for people with dementia."

Habilitation

For everyone with Alzheimer's, but especially those who've progressed from the mildest stages, a nationally recognized expert in the field has a wise and different way of treating afflicted loved ones in the home. She calls it "habilitation," and what it amounts to is a whole different approach for minimizing the stress of the disease on all concerned.

The expert is Joanne Koenig Coste, and her book is *Learning to Speak Alzheimer's*. If I can boil it down to a sentence, "habilitation" is about seeing Alzheimer's through the eyes of the loved one who has it, and making a lot of very profound changes, as a result, in the way the family treats her.

Take the all-too-common statement a loved one with Alzheimer's makes about her parents: that they're still alive, and she plans to see them soon. You know what the knee-jerk response is: "No they're not! They've been dead for years!" So jangled is the afflicted person—sheepish, confused, agitated—that she tends to react negatively, either declaring her family member has just told her a lie, or even lashing out physically. Why not instead respond by saying, gently, "Tell me what you love most about them." The patient is soothed, and what harm is done by this little white lie, if that's even what it is?

That's the essence of habilitation.

In her book, Joanne goes through all the daily rituals of home life with an afflicted person, and tweaks them through the lens of habilitation. Just putting the toothpaste on the toothbrush before he goes into the bathroom—and putting the razor next to the shaving cream—can make a loved one's ablutions easier to cope with for him. Putting the day's clothes out on the bed. Removing unnecessary utensils and other objects from the dining room table. More subtly, the "habilitator," as Joanne puts it, should keep an ear open for odd, recurrent sounds that may go unnoticed by everyone else but jar and perhaps upset the loved one with Alzheimer's. Putting dimmer switches on the lights, and turning them up as the afternoon light fades, may avoid the anxious hour of sundowning. Putting a black mat by the front door may subtly discourage the loved one from going out wandering. As the disease progresses, a person with Alzheimer's may be startled and alarmed by her image in a mirror, perhaps thinking she's seeing an intruder. Best, then, to remove the mirror—and furniture that may be hard to navigate.

At the same time, Joanne suggests some helpful additions. Childproofing extendable gates at the top and bottom of the stairs. Posters that show sun-filled, attractive destinations. Kill switches on the stove and other kitchen appliances that may cause harm. And outside: perhaps an herb garden that the loved one with Alzheimer's can savor and help maintain on summer days.

Joanne's book has far too many other wise words of advice to include here, but I'll quote just one more—a sentence that sums up the essence of habilitation as an alternative therapy. "Never attempt to reason with someone who has lost her reason." Instead, just do all you can to keep her happy and at peace.

Amen.

Herbal Medicine

Among other Western and Asian herbal medicines that have anecdotal effectiveness with dementia are Choto-san, which contains eleven medicinal plants; Kami-Umtan-To, a combination of thirteen different plants; and Yizhi Jiannao capsule—a Chinese traditional herbal medicine that has had some benefit with vascular dementia, and may work with Alzheimer's. The National Institute of Medical Herbalists is one source for more information; the Register of Chinese Herbal Medicine is another.

Marijuana

As a national debate swirls around the benefits of marijuana for alleviating pain in cancer and various neurological diseases, new evidence suggests that it may be effective in
blocking the formation of amyloid plaques. Last year, a research
team from the University of South Florida published its findings in the highly regarded *Journal of Alzheimer's Disease*. Its
conclusion: the chemical in marijuana known as THC appears
to slow the production of the beta-amyloid protein that forms
those plaques. Though scientists continue to argue whether the
plaques or tau tangles play the principal role in killing brain
cells, most scientists acknowledge that amyloid plaques play at
least a role. If THC can keep those plaques from forming, might
it actually be the cure for Alzheimer's? One of the study's authors cautions that more research is needed. Even if THC does
block plaque formation, it may not be safe for everyone: many
are the prospective miracle drugs that turn out to stop a disease while harming the patient. Howard, for one, is adamant: he
won't even consider prescribing marijuana to any patient unless
and until a whole lot more testing is done to confirm its safety
and efficacy—and determine that it has no adverse behavioral
effects. He's skeptical that marijuana will meet that threshold.

This is one of those possibilities that I put in the category
of promising for the future—but of no help for B. or any other
mid- to severe-stage Alzheimer's patients. Their plaques have
formed already; that ship has sailed. Still, it's a cheering report, maybe the most cheering I've heard about yet. And the
study's success has that Florida team now trying the cocktail
approach—putting THC in with caffeine and other natural

compounds that might slow the growth of those plaques. The cocktail approach is what made AIDS a manageable disease. Maybe it's the answer for Alzheimer's, too.

Massage

Though no scientific studies affirm the therapeutic value of massage, anecdotal experience—and common sense—suggest that it can alleviate anxiety, agitation, and depression.

Meditation and Yoga

A study done at Beth Israel Deaconess Medical Center in Boston divided a group of fourteen adults between the ages of fifty-five and ninety. One group was given regular care but no meditation or yoga; the other was given the same care but practiced yoga and meditation at least two hours a week. The latter group had less brain atrophy, especially in the memory-central hippocampus, and better brain connectivity.

Again, no guarantees, but meditation is given credit for everything from diminishing stress in Alzheimer's patients to lessening the sense of social isolation that many feel. It's said to reduce the stress hormone cortisol, associated with the risk of developing dementia.

Bottom line: there is nothing bad about meditating, and maybe a lot of good. B. and I haven't done it ourselves yet, but it's on our short list for 2015, and the Hamptons have so many yoga options that it's hard to avoid them!

Music Therapy

Again, no scientific proof exists to support it, but music therapy appears to ease the anxiety and agitation in Alzheimer's patients. Soothing music that the patient likes may, if played for at least half an hour for the patient in an otherwise quiet room, have the same effects it has on the rest of us!

TENS

A mild electrical current is relayed through electrodes stuck to the skin, in the process called TENS, but more formally known as transcutaneous electrical nerve stimulation. It may cause a slight prickling feeling, but it is not at all painful—and indeed is used to alleviate pain, often with women in labor. Again, there's no proof that it eases anxiety and agitation in Alzheimer's patients, but there is some anecdotal suggestion that it may.

PART 9

ALZHEIMER'S AND AFRICAN AMERICANS

As far as home-care help goes, I don't really need someone. I know better than to get in my car and go somewhere. And walking is no problem—I just walk down the beach into Sag Harbor. Usually I don't even get beyond the dog run down the beach. I let Bishop run with the other dogs, and chitchat with the other dog owners. Why do I need someone guarding me for that?

I can understand why Dan would want somebody to come in. For things as simple as forgetting that I took something from here and put it over there. Those are the little things that aren't that little. They usually turn out to be big.

What I don't need is someone to sort out my clothes closet for me. Dan keeps bugging me about it, until he finally hired this young woman to do it. I don't want her coming. It's my closet. I do my closet my way.

There are other rules Dan has put on me. Like no more driving. No more driving! That's hard. I've been driving since I was a teenager—and that white Mercedes sports coupe in the driveway was a gift to me. "You can't drive anymore, B.," says Dan. "No driving for you." I get angry, but I know he's right. I'm not going to fight that one. I'm not crazy! Just a little here and there.

One thing I haven't lost is my sense of humor. You can't lose that!

Lately, I've been thinking a lot about going home; have I mentioned that? I think I'll wait until Mother's Day to go. I want to see the house, and my old room. I want to see if the fruit trees are still there, and the grape arbor. I want to see if my mother's put flowers out, and taste her pineapple upside-down cake again. In my whole life I've never tasted anything so good as her pineapple upside-down cake.

There was a little soda shop in Everson where we went after school; I want to see if that's still there. I want to take the bridge over to Scottdale and go to that clothing store that loaned me clothes when I was going to modeling school. They were awfully nice to me there. And then I want to come back to the house, and smell dinner on the stove, and feel that wonderful feeling of being home again.

TWENTY-NINE

NEW YORK CITY

Fall 2014

I was fascinated—and appalled—that Alzheimer's claimed so many African Americans. It was like this secret hidden in plain sight. And so I set out to make some sense of it all.

Back in the 1980s, as scientists started sequencing genes, they noted intriguing disparities between the genes in white and black Americans. One of those, APOE-e4, appeared to be more prevalent in blacks than whites: "overexpressed," as the scientists put it. And that was intriguing, because the proportion of African Americans who get Alzheimer's is greater than that of whites—up to 100 percent more. (In sheer numbers, of course, fewer blacks get Alzheimer's than whites because there are fewer of them: they constitute about 14 percent of the US population. It's the proportional disparity that's so dramatic and troubling.) Maybe APOE-e4 became more damaging in tandem with some other gene in African Americans. Or maybe lifestyle-related factors increased the chance that APOE-e4 would start the process of forming amyloid plaques and tau tangles.

Back in 2002, Dr. Goldie Byrd, a biologist, did a sabbatical year at Duke University and got a close look at a research trial under way to learn more about the genetics of Alzheimer's. In particular, the researchers were trying to understand the high incidence of Alzheimer's among African Americans, but Dr. Byrd could see they didn't have a prayer—not when only 43 of their 7,000 blood samples were from African Americans.

The researchers weren't biased or careless. They were just up against decades of mistrust in the black community that came down to one word: *Tuskegee.* It was a word I knew well. Beginning in the early 1930s, federal researchers had enrolled six hundred poor Alabama sharecroppers in a long-term study of their "bad blood," ostensibly to restore them to health. What the researchers meant by "bad blood" was syphilis. The sharecroppers weren't told that most had the disease in its early stages, and that the study, based at the Tuskegee Institute, was being done to see how it would play out among them. Worse, when penicillin was proven by the late 1940s to eradicate syphilis, the sharecroppers weren't given it. Not until word of the experiment leaked to the press in 1972 did the Tuskegee Syphilis Study get shut down. By then many men in the study had died; others had infected their wives; and children had been born with congenital syphilis. The study went down as the most glaring breach of bioethics in American history.

That was the history the Duke researchers were up against in 2002. It didn't help that most of them were white.

Another visiting scientist at Duke, Margaret Pericak-Vance of the University of Miami, urged Dr. Byrd to start up a trial of her own, back at North Carolina A&T State University, where Goldie was a professor. The two ended up working together;

they're research partners still, and what they've built is unique: the first major Alzheimer's research trial for African Americans in the United States.

"It was very helpful that we were in a historical black university, right in the middle of a big black community," Dr. Byrd told me. Also that the lead investigator—Dr. Byrd herself—was black.

The trial was for African Americans already diagnosed with Alzheimer's. It was just a research trial: no new drugs, just tracking the participants as their illness progressed. Many were too sick when the trial began to make up their own minds about whether to join; their caregivers had to decide for them. Before making that request, Goldie embarked on a listening tour of black communities. "What are your barriers?" she asked caregivers. "What do you need from us even after we ascertain that your loved one would qualify for the study?"

Tuskegee came up a lot. "It wasn't the most sensitive thing," Goldie told me. "People remembered that, but the most important thing was that they didn't want their loved ones to be guinea pigs, used and abandoned." That was a widespread fear even though this wasn't a drug trial. Dr. Byrd and her team would just be studying their volunteers' blood and tracking their cognitive decline. The point wasn't to come up with a new miracle drug. It was to learn how Alzheimer's affected African Americans—and ultimately, why such a higher proportion of blacks than whites got the disease. Eventually, many respondents came to view their loved ones' involvement as a civic responsibility. "When they said they'd be in the study," Dr. Byrd said, "they followed through."

Goldie started with about 1,000 participants. By 2013, she

and Pericak-Vance had joined forces with a national consortium of researchers, headed by Dr. Richard Mayeux of Columbia University, studying nearly 6,000 African Americans sixty years or older. Some had Alzheimer's; others, the "control" participants, did not. No one had ever done a trial of this scope on the subject. The scientific goal: to determine whether certain genes put blacks at greater risk for Alzheimer's than that of whites of European ancestry.

The consortium's report, published in 2013, was both tantalizing and frustrating. It turned out that African Americans with Alzheimer's are slightly more likely than whites to have a certain gene known as ABCA7, which in turn makes them somewhat more apt to get Alzheimer's. But ABCA7 is relatively rare, so that even if the study suggested a clear cause and effect—which it didn't—that would still leave 90 percent of Alzheimer's in African Americans unexplained. As for the original bad actor, APOE-e4, it was found as often in whites as in African Americans. So it, too, failed to explain why so many more African Americans than whites get Alzheimer's. But this, as Dr. Byrd reminded me, is how medical science advances: as often by ruling out theories as by ruling them in.

While Dr. Byrd works toward understanding the complex factors that lead to Alzheimer's in African Americans, she's already done something quite remarkable. She's helped her whole community to get over the stigma of Alzheimer's by doing the kind of outreach that all of us should support. As dean of arts and sciences at North Carolina A&T State University, she's missed no chance to get out the word about it: to promote early testing and diagnosis, and get help for families struggling with the disease. She and her staffers and volunteers have done galas and auctions, sponsored conferences and fund-raising walks, gone to churches to get clergy and congregation to wear Alzheimer's purple for raising awareness, staged town hall meetings and workshops, recruited the football team and cheerleaders to wave purple plumes, and flashed Alzheimer's awareness messages on the stadium's Jumbotron screen. Probably her most important outreach effort has come in response to what caregivers told her they needed most: support groups.

Imagine every town and city in America waving the Alzheimer's purple, staging awareness and fund-raising events, knocking the stigma out of this awful disease, getting people tested sooner, and rallying everyone to join a research or clinical trial—because without volunteers, there will *be* no new drugs, and we'll still be fighting a losing battle.

Last November, Dr. Byrd took her outreach operation one giant step further. With a $1 million grant from the pharmaceutical company Merck, she turned a 3,100-square-foot building into what she calls COAACH: the Center for Outreach in Alzheimer's, Aging, and Community Health. It helps both patients and caregivers, links them as needed to the national Alzheimer's Association—and basically does the home-care piece that doctors can't afford to do. Hearing about what's going on down at North Carolina A&T gives me hope—and with Alzheimer's, that's a damned good thing to feel.

A long with all these efforts, Dr. Goldie Byrd has helped found a national group called the African American Network Against Alzheimer's. There's some serious money behind it, and a lot of that comes from an unexpected source: a white former corporate lawyer named George Vradenburg, and his wife, Trish.

George was chief counsel at America Online and CBS, as well as a senior executive at AOL Time Warner and the Fox Broadcasting company. He might have retired to a life of yachting and golf. But George, like so many people who take up the fight against Alzheimer's, had a personal motivation: his mother-in-law died of it. Trish was a highly successful television writer—for the show *Designing Women*—when that happened. She wrote a play about the impact of her mother's illness on her whole family. The play was called *Surviving Grace*. Soon the Vradenburgs were hosting galas in Washington for the Alzheimer's Association. By 2010, George and Trish had made Alzheimer's their full-time cause. They formed a national group called USAgainstAlzheimer's, an umbrella with various subgroups under it. One of those is the African American Network Against Alzheimer's.

George and Trish are committed to helping back clinical research that leads to new breakthroughs in treatment. But they're also focused on the home-care side. Last year, USAgainstAlzheimer's funded the first major study of the cost of Alzheimer's for black Americans. Its conclusions are shocking. Despite making up that modest 14 percent of the national population, blacks bear 30 percent of the costs of Alzheimer's. In 2012, that came out to $71.6 billion of the roughly $215 billion overall cost to US families. Most of that money, the study found, was for caregivers. A lot of it was money paid to home health-care workers; much of the rest was counted as wages lost by family caregivers forced to cut back on or quit their jobs. The bulk of that $71.6 billion was spent in the southern states, where a black American's odds of getting Alzheimer's between the ages of 75 and 84 are at 1 in 3, and 1 in 2 by the age of 85. By 2050, the study's authors predict, those costs will double as the number of blacks in old age soars.

Along with crunching the numbers, the study offers several hypotheses for why the incidence of Alzheimer's among aging African Americans seems so much higher than that of whites. Along with whatever the gene story turns out to be, the study's authors suggest that poor education may be one contributing factor, poor diet another. Those factors act to slow cognitive development; they literally slow growth of the brain. How unlikely is it then that late in life, an undernourished brain may be less able to ward off the amyloid plaques and tau tangles that lead to Alzheimer's?

Environmental factors may also play a role. African Americans in the rural South often work amid dangerous toxins, from heavy metals to pesticides; the study's authors suspect that physical stresses like these make a difference, too. For that matter, they theorize, the stress of poverty, exacerbated by racism and its own, unremitting psychological pressure, may help bring on Alzheimer's for African Americans. Is it by chance that the incidence of Alzheimer's for African Americans is highest in the rural South, where all these factors are at their highest? "I know everyone is skeptical about whether these are major factors," Dr. Byrd told me. "But I do believe that socioeconomics contributes to health disparities."

Dr. Byrd isn't the only expert to harbor this suspicion. "In typical late-onset Alzheimer's," says Dr. John Hardy of the National Institute on Aging in a recent documentary on Alzheimer's for HBO, "we know it isn't a simple mutation. We expect it to be a mix of causes, of predispositions, some environmental and some genetic." Hardy talks of "susceptibility genes" that may increase the risk of Alzheimer's in various ways. Add a lifetime of poverty, debilitating work, and institutional racism, and the odds seem to shoot straight up—to diabetes, hypertension, vascular disease, and ultimately to Alzheimer's.

Sorting out the exact roles that genetics, socioeconomics, and environment play in Alzheimer's—and how each affects the other—may be the work of generations to come. Here's one thing we know for sure, though: whatever role genes turn out to play in Alzheimer's, our understanding will owe a lot to a poor black woman from Roanoke, Virginia, who grew up in a log cabin once used as slave quarters. In the unspooling history of Alzheimer's and African Americans, one of the most significant figures is clearly Henrietta Lacks.

For most of her short life, nothing about Henrietta Lacks seemed likely to land her in the history of science. Born in 1920, she seemed healthy until the onset of a pain that turned out to be cervical cancer. At just thirty, with her symptoms worsening, Henrietta went to Johns Hopkins Hospital, where her doctor noticed that blood cells in her cervical tumor appeared to be outliving normal cells that typically lasted just a few days. Not only that: these unusual cells kept replicating in the petri dish. Doctors had never seen cells do that before. Their durability and powers of multiplication made them unique—and, in a sense, immortal.

Henrietta died soon after, but her cells kept replicating in petri dishes, and living long enough to be useful in a wide range of biomedical experiments. With them, Dr. Jonas Salk developed the polio vaccine. HeLa cells, as they became known, in a nod to their late donor's first and last names, were put to use in cancer research, gene mapping, in vitro fertilization—and, yes, Alzheimer's research. HeLa cells have been used in some seventy thousand medical studies, and counting.

Henrietta was never informed that her cells had been harvested and put into the service of medical science. Nor was her family, which remained poor while Henrietta's unique cells lived on, making possible billion-dollar drugs and countless research advances. In 2010, Henrietta's story was told in the best-selling *The Immortal Life of Henrietta Lacks,* by Rebecca Skloot. The book raised important ethical questions about how doctors should have handled HeLa cells all along. Shouldn't they have sought Henrietta's permission, and later her family's, before using her cells? Didn't her family have a right to say how, and when, HeLa cells could be used at all? And given that HeLa cells led to billion-dollar drugs, shouldn't the family get some sort of compensation?

The debate was still reverberating in 2013 when Henrietta's genome was sequenced—and published—by doctors who seemed oblivious to the trammeling of privacy rights for Henrietta's descendants. By doing so, the doctors made public any and all genetic predispositions that Lacks family members had—to cancer, to bipolar disorder, and, yes, to Alzheimer's—possibly stigmatizing them, even costing them jobs. Only then did the National Institutes of Health establish a clear protocol on how HeLa cells would be used from now on—by asking the Lacks family for permission.

HeLa cells haven't yet led to the biomedical explanation for how Alzheimer's begins and progresses. But almost certainly, when those explanations come, HeLa cells will have made that research possible. It's quite a legacy already for a black Virginian woman whose family couldn't even afford medical insurance—and a reminder that with Alzheimer's, we're all in this together: black and white. It's the prisoner's dilemma: two prisoners, manacled to each other, hoping to break out of jail. Neither one can do it without the other: if they're going to make a break for it, they have to make it out—in step—together.

I was thrilled to learn that the campaign to get more African Americans into Alzheimer's trials has an unofficial leader in the country's most distinguished African American doctor: David Satcher.

Back in the mid-1990s, as director of the US Centers for Disease Control and Prevention, Dr. Satcher took a step toward redressing the overall problem of so few African Americans in drug trials of every kind. The nation needed to come to terms with the bitter legacy of Tuskegee. "I put together a commission," he explained to me, "to see if we could put it behind us."

Dr. Satcher showed the commission's findings to President Clinton, who immediately agreed there should be a presidential apology, which he proceeded to issue on May 16, 1997. "I think seven of the participants were alive; they were there," Satcher recalled. "But this wasn't just an empty apology." With it went a new bioethics center at Tuskegee where physicians and researchers could be trained in ethics research. Also, the president decreed, from now on the community in which a research trial was held would have to be involved from start to finish. (Henrietta Lacks's genome was published by a research team based in Heidelberg, Germany, outside the pale of these new US guidelines.)

So in fact, there wouldn't—couldn't—ever be another Tuskegee, at least not in the United States. "But as you know, things get really clouded when it comes to race in this country," Dr. Satcher observed, "so it's not easy to put Tuskegee behind us."

Dr. Satcher, who went on to serve as the country's sixteenth surgeon general in the last two years of Clinton's presidency and the first two years of George W. Bush's, thinks the key to bringing African Americans into drug trials is getting their physicians involved. "People listen to their doctors," Dr. Satcher noted. The more black doctors who urge their patients, with or without Alzheimer's, to join research and clinical trials, the sooner those trials will have the 20 percent black volunteers they need. That, in turn, will lead to results that help explain why more African Americans get Alzheimer's—and what drugs, in what dosages, are right for them.

As surgeon general, Dr. Satcher had the military rank of admiral, and the fancy uniform to go with it, set off with gold braid. At seventy-three, he's still a striking figure with a public health message: that African Americans bear an undue burden of vascular disease, diabetes, and hypertension, as well as the four leading kinds of cancer: lung, prostate, colorectal, and breast. Genetics is part of it, but so, he's convinced, are all those socioeconomic factors in the home, school, and workplace, from poor education to malnutrition to toxic substances that surround factory workers. Dr. Satcher feels sure that some if not all of those chronic diseases lead to Alzheimer's, and he's still doing all he can to get the word out, to raise both funding and awareness. Last year, he joined George Vradenburg and Dr. Goldie Byrd and about a dozen others in founding the African American Network Against Alzheimer's.

"We're way behind on research," Dr. Satcher laments. "We need so much more federal funding, especially to address the high morbidity of African Americans from Alzheimer's. And what do we do about that? Washington is so dysfunctional now. I remember when you could really organize and reason with people in the House and the Senate. Everything is so political now, it's hard to get something done. If Obama proposes, you can bet on the Republican majority being against it. We just have to keep pushing, and educating, and building pressure for more research." Ironically, as more and more American families struggle with Alzheimer's, Dr. Satcher feels sure that pressure will build. "The burden of caregiving is so severe," Dr. Satcher says with a sigh, "I know that most families can't afford it. It saddens me that people are quitting their jobs to tend their sick parents or spouses."

As a veteran viewer of the big picture, Dr. Satcher is especially frustrated these days by the contrast between funding for Alzheimer's and the big bundle of federal money for Ebola. With the recent scare, he observes, the politicians went wildly overboard, responding to irrational public fears. The Obama administration went so far as to request $6 *billion* from Congress for Ebola prevention. "That's more than the federal government has spent on Alzheimer's research over the entirety of the last decade," Dr. Satcher exclaims. And for what? "So far there have been four US cases of Ebola and two deaths. And while every death is tragic, an estimated five hundred thousand Americans will die this year because they have Alzheimer's."

Admittedly, Alzheimer's is not contagious. "However," Dr. Satcher says, "because it is driven by age-related demographics, its impact will grow as if it were. The number of Americans with Alzheimer's will grow from more than five million today to as many as sixteen million by midcentury. Caring for people with Alzheimer's will cost our country trillions in today's dollars over this same period.

"If you happen to be more frightened by Ebola than by Alzheimer's," Dr. Satcher adds, "consider this. While there is virtually no chance of contracting Ebola in the US right now, the likelihood of developing Alzheimer's or needing to care for someone with Alzheimer's is staggering. Thankfully, some who have developed Ebola have survived. No one has yet survived Alzheimer's.

"The bottom line on the big picture is this," Dr. Satcher says. "Alzheimer's is the most underrecognized threat to public health in the twenty-first century. If we have the resources to address Ebola, we have them for Alzheimer's, too. It's time to bring Alzheimer's to the front of our agenda."

As is the case for so many of the scientists and researchers working on Alzheimer's, Dr. Satcher's involvement is both professional and keenly personal: for more than a decade, he's been the caregiver to his wife, Nola.

Long before Nola was diagnosed, the Satchers knew that her odds weren't good: her mother came down with early-onset Alzheimer's in her early sixties. Nola's mother lived until ninety-three but spent her last fifteen years in an institution. Nola got her own diagnosis at about the same age her mother did.

Nola is still living at home, a tribute both to her strength of spirit—and to her family's means. "She would not be at home if we didn't have the resources and the family we have," Dr. Satcher explains.

Nola was a poet, which makes her loss of language especially cruel. Until a year ago, she could recite long stretches of poetry, both others' and her own. "Music, singing, poetry—they tend to endure longer than other things," Dr. Satcher observes. "What is it about rhyme and music and poetry? Maybe the brain stores them somewhere safe as long as it can. My wife still remembers the words to songs in church."

Dr. Satcher had heard about B.'s disappearance, and offered comforting words about that. "Nola went through the stage of walking off, too," he told me. "That went on a couple years. You had to be quite aware of her moves; she was found walking out in the streets. But then she stopped, and we haven't had that problem for quite a while."

I asked if after all these years tending her, Dr. Satcher still had some semblance of a marriage with Nola, or if by now he was relegated solely to the roles of companion and caregiver. That was probably too personal a question, but the doctor took no offense. "We do have a meaningful relationship," he said. "But it waxes and wanes. There are times, more now than even three months ago, where she will say, 'What's your name?' If I say, 'What do you think my name is?' she'll usually figure it out. Still, almost every day, she says, 'I love you.' "

LESSONS LEARNED

A Story of Two States

If there's one thing I've learned about fighting back against Alzheimer's, it's that none of us can do it alone. We can't deal with one case of it alone; we certainly can't hope to make progress against it as a disease without a sustained campaign linking caregivers and home-based health workers, nonprofits and educational groups, doctors and scientists and professors, policy makers and politicians, church leaders and federal agencies, drug companies and medical venture capitalists—and let's not forget book writers, and journalists and playwrights and filmmakers. Here's another, simpler way to put it: we need individuals, and we need communities. The good news is that all these efforts are giving rise to new, vigorous community groups—groups that are helping patients and caregivers, getting out the word, and building the power for change. Our current president began as a community organizer. With faith and persistence, there's no better way to build consensus and make things happen. One of the states that illustrates that is North Carolina, where Dr. Goldie Byrd has helped make the Center for Outreach in Alzheimer's, Aging, and Community Health (COAACH) a driving force. The other is Minnesota.

In 2009, the Minnesota legislature declared enough was enough: Minnesotans with Alzheimer's needed help, and so did their families. Recommendations were drawn up, and two years later, ACT on Alzheimer's was established as a statewide network of volunteer stakeholders: medical, academic, business, and nonprofit, all dedicated to implementing those recommendations.

A lot of good initiatives soon fizzle out. Not ACT on Alzheimer's. Look at the state map on its website (www.actonalz .org). Thirty-three communities from International Falls down to Harmony are red-dotted on that map. Click on the dots and feel the civic dedication radiating out from your screen. In Walker, for example, volunteers are heartily putting their 2013 action plan into gear. One of their two top priorities is resource access. "A common thread throughout our survey process was that people didn't know where to go for resources about Alzheimer's and dementia," explains Melanie Deegan, Walker's team leader, "so we want to educate about accessing resources." That starts with encouraging Minnesotans to get early diagnosis and quality care, memory-loss services, emergency preparedness, and response—in short, all the stuff I wish that B. and I had had three years ago in the heart of New York City.

Priority two for the Walker volunteers is educating the Chamber of Commerce and local merchants about Alzheimer's, and creating dementia-friendly stores and municipal services. Businesses that participate in a simple training course will get a dementia-friendly logo they can put on their store window.

The recent movie *Still Alice,* starring Julianne Moore, portrays a fifty-year-old woman's descent into early Alzheimer's. Socially it has been a huge help in educating communities about Alzheimer's and—hopefully—lessening the stigma of the disease. At ACT on Alzheimer's, not surprisingly, the movie and the book on which it was based have been used statewide as educational tools—all part of an ongoing campaign that includes everything from training local emergency responders to working with rabbis to creating memory cafés.

As far as I can tell, Minnesota is way ahead of most states in education and activism on Alzheimer's, right up there with North Carolina. We need the other forty-eight to catch up.

PART 10

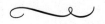

THE ROAD AHEAD

It's going to be interesting, going through this next year. Whatever happens in this year is the future. What has been given to me has been given to me. It's not the worst thing. It's a lifestyle that's totally changed. But I'm alive. I can take my meds. I don't feel shortchanged. I want to continue to be the best I can be. And keep on living.

I like it here in Sag Harbor, but if I'm going to continue to do things, I have to do them in the city. I want to get back in play.

If I had to choose one thing to get involved in, it would be Alzheimer's. The restaurant—I don't love the business enough anymore. But I have to figure out what I'm going to do. I'm not going to just hang around.

One thought is about singing. At one point in my life it was a serious ambition. I worked up a repertoire of standards I liked, and had a backup trio, and performed at a place called the Briars on the Upper West Side. At another point I was a singer with a band—more contemporary, I guess you'd say. I got a lot of compliments, and not just from my friends. From other club owners, too. But unless you land a record deal, singing in clubs just sort of dribbles along. In the end I saw that my best hope was modeling, and then starting my own restaurant after that. And then it was

Dan who came in and saw the potential to make me more widely known, and make a national business of it. I owe him so much. And now that I'm sick, I don't know how I'm going to keep on doing the things that made it all work.

But I'm still serious about singing. Just because you have Alzheimer's doesn't mean you can't sing. Especially when they have those karaoke screens with the lyrics on them. And when you get people singing with you, it helps. It gets you moving and thinking, and even if you do something that's a little bit off, you just put the song back on. I'm not going to forget the tunes I love, that's for sure. I'll remember those tunes my whole life. So that's my plan, and I'm sticking to it! I'm going to work for Alzheimer's, and I'm going to sing, maybe even at a club or two again. With those karaoke screens, you can't really forget the words, they're right in front of you.

And then all you have to do is sing.

THIRTY

SAG HARBOR

Winter 2014–2015

Last week I took action at last—on B.'s great mess of a clothes closet. I hired a young woman to come in and organize it. Now it looks as it once did: all the dresses neatly hung, the shoes in neat rows. It stuns me to see such order restored. It's like going back in time. Now if only I could pay someone to do that for B.'s mind.

I hired that young woman while B. was still feeling contrite about wandering all night and scaring the bejesus out of everyone who loves her. I saw my chance and took it. Victory! Until B. came to inspect the difference. "I don't need some stranger to tell me how to hang my clothes," she huffed. "How dare she."

I hadn't expected anything different. Nor were my feelings hurt—not at this stage in the game. We caregivers know: not only does no good deed go unpunished, it gets forgotten, too! You don't get a thank-you when a person has Alzheimer's. You can't expect them to appreciate all the things you do for them.

They'll rarely say thank you, because it's not on their screen. Which is draining. At the end of the day, you want to be appreciated for what you do each day by the people who love you. That's human. To know that is something you'll never get . . . it's hard. But still we go on, day after day, because really, what choice do we have?

No, that's not quite true. Home-care help—that's a choice. Until, you might say, it's no longer a choice: you have to have it. B. and I are clearly to that point—beyond it, as far as our doctor is concerned. I keep interviewing prospects; B. keeps shooting them down. I know I should just bring someone in no matter what B. says. Somehow I just can't do that. Not quite yet.

Christmas is coming, and for the first time in our twenty-two years together, we've gotten an artificial tree. We love the real ones, but I just realized we can't take the chance. What if B. lights a candle beside the tree while I'm down at the beach walking Bishop? The whole house could go up in flames. I didn't think this way before the Very Bad Night, but now I do: we've entered a new stage. Or maybe we entered it months ago and I just didn't accept it.

In this new stage—Stage Five by the seven-stage model, Stage Two by the three-stage model—I not only can't leave B. alone in the house for long, but I have to treat her the way I would a puppy. You love that puppy, but you know you can't trust her on her own for a minute. Before you know it, your adorable puppy will pull the Christmas tree down.

This morning we worked together, putting the artificial branches into the metal pole trunk. It made for a good activity, and B. took pride in sticking in her share of branches. This afternoon we brought up the tree ornaments from the basement, cranked up the Nat King Cole Christmas album, and hung them on the tree. The ornaments have stories, going back as far as Everson, Pennsylvania. Last year B. recalled most of those stories. This year, not as many.

I know and accept that B. is now in midstage Alzheimer's. Yet in so many ways she's still B. Which is to say that so far, she doesn't exhibit most of the symptoms associated with Stage Two—or Stage Five, whatever you want to call it. She's still warm and affectionate most of the time; when she does get angry or agitated, it passes. She sticks to a healthy diet, takes long walks on the beach with Bishop, even goes to the gym now to work out with our trainer. Physically she's still strong—powerful, even. Remember, this is a woman who walked the streets of Manhattan for seventeen hours—in high heels! Historically, standing armies moved twenty miles a day—that was as far as they could go before they got so tired they couldn't fight. B. had to have gone at least that far that night and next day.

Typically, in the middle stages, other signs of difference—big signs—start to appear. B. hasn't exhibited those yet. Loss of coordination—hand tremors, sloppier handwriting, trouble managing zippers or buttons, an unsteady walk? Not B. Trouble getting out of bed or a chair? No way. Trouble bathing or dressing? Not at all. Messy eating, trouble swallowing, hoarding of food in the bedroom? No, no, and no. Failure to recognize familiar faces? No more than the rest of us do. Clinging to her caregiver, following me around? If anything, the opposite! The symptoms she does have, worse at night—sundowning, as doctors call it? No, except . . . B. did wander off from that jitney at dusk. Some would call that sundowning.

I know the symptoms B. has—the short-term memory loss, the closet-rummaging and wanting to go "home," and all the rest. I just want to believe that B. remains near the start of that middle stage. If so, she may have quite a few more years of relative mobility, human dignity, and simple pleasures. She may actually be happy much of that time—and if she's happy, I can live with that. Assuming we get home-care help—and that's just a matter of when, not if—maybe four days a week, I can envision a not-too-bad state of affairs where I go into the city two or three of those days for work while B. is cared for, and spend the rest of the week at home in what you might call harmony. Okay—maybe not three- or four-part harmony but a peaceful coexistence with the woman I love, whose spirit remains, to some extent, intact.

Of course, I may be in denial here: bargaining again with Alzheimer's, a disease that is, I have come to see, completely merciless. Maybe it's killing B.'s brain cells at a faster rate than expected, moving relentlessly toward her frontal lobes. Maybe she's really somewhere in the middle of that middle-to-severe stage. Howard hasn't said that exactly, but I know he's troubled by those cognitive tests he gave B. not long ago.

Here's why I think I'm not in denial: I know what happens in the final stage, and I know, barring some new drug's miraculous arrival, that that's where B. is heading. I didn't think that a year ago. I thought we'd hang on until the new drug came along, and beat this thing after all. I'm still optimistic—but more for others than for us. The drugs *will* come, and a next generation may not have to endure this terrible ordeal. I just have to be realistic now about the chances of saving B.

Being realistic means more than expecting the situation to

get worse. It means taking in the details of what will happen, and making appropriate plans.

In the late stage, as I now understand, amyloid plaques spread throughout the brain, like so many tombstones, accompanied by the so-called tau tangles associated with dead brain cells. The only part of the brain left intact is the strip of motor cortex and visual cortex. That's why hospital-bound patients with end-stage Alzheimer's do much walking and pacing: it's the last thing they know how to do.

With the onset of the severe stage, a loved one loses the ability to communicate, along with the most basic social skills. That may bring on bursts of rage and profanity. It may bring violence, too, as a frustrated patient lashes out against her caregiver by smacking him. Just as likely, severe-stage Alzheimer's may leave the patient docile or apathetic for long periods. She's no longer capable of sequential thought, or of any tasks involving it: apathy is the giving up of her effort to think.

In the severe stage, language begins to fall away. The patient may not understand what you say; she may not have the words to respond. She may withdraw from social interactions. She may lose her sense of self. Now even long-term memory starts to fade.

A patient with severe-stage Alzheimer's needs more than the company of a home-care worker. She needs help with basic functions: bathing, dressing, eating, and, eventually, what the literature discreetly calls toileting. Likely that means moving her into an assisted-living center, where she can get as much help as she needs.

Last to go are the senses and basic mobility. Talking gently and lovingly to a patient is helpful. So is touching her cheek and giving her a hug. These are gestures she likely still understands. Taking her into the sunshine, feeling a warm breeze, maybe watching a squirrel—these are the last of the simple pleasures to go.

At some point, a patient will lose even the ability to walk, and so become bedridden, as the motor and visual cortex go, too. Now the focus is on trying to keep her from developing pressure sores, on dealing with incontinence, on keeping her fed and hydrated. Let's be blunt: in end-stage Alzheimer's, the patient is basically immobile, incommunicative, and unresponsive, and death is imminent as one organ after another shuts down. The literature has only these words of comfort for a patient and her family at this stage. Remember, there is still a living spirit inside this diminished person, the spirit of someone you love.

So there: I see it. I see it all. But if, as we hope, B. remains near the start of that mid-to-severe stage, then we have six, maybe eight, maybe ten years left of midrange coping, and there's a lot we can do with that.

First, as a family, we can spend more time together. B. loves it when Dana is with us, and Dana loves being with her mom. Now Dana brings Sansa, her puppy, and B. lights up as soon as she sees him. Bishop gets in on the hugs and kisses, too, and we spend hours at a time playing with the two of those dogs and watching them interact.

That's the way we spent our Christmas, with a lot of Christmas joy, out here in Sag Harbor. The celebration started two days before, because that's our wedding anniversary: our twenty-second. All those twenty-two years later, I'm still B.'s cut man in the corner, and to the extent she can be, she's mine. I didn't expect to be spending the holiday filling out B.'s Social Security and Medicare forms, but as Alzheimer's-related tasks go, that's a relatively happy one.

Meanwhile, I'm thrilled to report that B. and I have found—at last!—a home health-care worker we both like. Isabel's from Ecuador, a lovely, joyous woman but not *too* young or attractive! Though she is, like B., beautiful inside and out. She's got experience of the kind you want even as you wince at the thought: she comes to us having just cared for an Alzheimer's patient who died. Well, that's the reality. We might as well face it. I'm just so relieved that she and B. get along so well, and that she's such an unobtrusive presence. We're going to start by having her at the house three days a week and see how that goes. At the least, I'll be able to go to the city for business without leaving B. on her own—a stage I know we reached some months ago, though we slid along in denial for too long after that. I can't tell you how much better that feels: all that guilt and anxiety lifted from my shoulders. Facing reality doesn't solve the problem. But it does make the reality easier to bear.

THIRTY-ONE

SAG HARBOR

Fall 2014

There's more we want to do, though, than bide our time at home. Almost every day, we get media requests for interviews with B. and me. We knew that B. was a national figure; we didn't anticipate that her illness would stir such interest and concern across the country, so much that the story just keeps reverberating. Partly, it's B. People feel they know her, and in a way they do: the still-warm, still-gracious woman they see on TV *is* B., and audiences can feel that glow as much as I do. Partly, it's the families of those 5.2 million Americans who have Alzheimer's, and the millions more of their friends and relatives. I believe they take comfort from B.'s courage in confronting this awful disease. At the same time, I think the audience is wider even than that. Let's face it: we're all terrified of getting this disease, and with every name or fact we forget, we feel a little stab of fear. Maybe we, too, we think, are destined to get Alzheimer's.

I want to turn that fear into positive action, as we've done with ours.

Here's my hit list so far:

Awareness

B. and I want to do all we can to make people aware of Alzheimer's early symptoms: those little signs of difference that so often get misinterpreted by families as marital tensions, or irascibility for no reason on the part of a parent or loved one. Knowing that those signs may denote Alzheimer's isn't terribly reassuring, but ultimately it's better to know than not and it can make a difference to treatment.

Seeking Medical Help Sooner Rather than Later

The doctors can't stress this enough: acting on those little signs instead of sweeping them under the rug is the best possible thing you can do. Fear keeps all too many of us from seeking medical help—and for those who do have Alzheimer's, it only allows the symptoms to grow worse. The two existing classes of Alzheimer's drugs are feeble, but to the extent they work, they seem to do so with patients who don't yet have the disease, only its precursor symptoms.

Getting a PET Imaging Diagnosis

This is a message we'll be beating the drum about again and again and again. The PET screen for amyloid plaques is a hugely important new tool in the fight against Alzheimer's. It's not a treatment and it's not a cure, but knowing for sure whether or not you have the disease—or, to be technical, whether you have the amyloid plaques associated with the disease—is a big step forward. For many who have Alzheimer's-like symptoms, it may bring absolution: a plaque-free PET screen. In that case a patient can know those little signs of difference are just normal signs of aging. Howard got a call not long ago from the wife and children of an eighty-two-year-old chairman and CEO of some major company. The chairman was having his lapses, at home and at work, and had begun to plan for his retirement. Almost as an afterthought—sure, as he was, that he did have Alzheimer's—the chairman got a PET imaging scan. He was amyloid-plaque free. With that, he could notify his board he'd be staying on another two or three years. Coincidence or not, he felt his memory sharpen overnight.

For those whose screens show these plaques, but not many as of yet, the test can be a wake-up call to start a lifestyle regimen— good diet and vigorous daily exercise—as well as the drugs. The cost of PET imaging is considerable—about five thousand dollars—and Medicare shows no sign of planning to cover it. Result: as many as 20–30 percent of Americans who *would* test positive for Alzheimer's or some other form of dementia don't get diagnosed. That's why we're supporting the Hope for Alzheimer's Act, more fully called the Health Outcomes, Planning, and Education (HOPE) for Alzheimer's Act. It calls for Medicare coverage not only of PET imaging but of care planning, both for the patient and caregiver.

To Howard Fillit, our doctor, an even more exciting development in screening is "imaging agents" that target the tangles— clumps of tau—that invariably appear with dying brain cells and may, as a result, be as good or better an indicator of Alzheimer's than the amyloid plaque screen. Amyloid plaques, as Howard observes, can be present in individuals who never develop symptoms of Alzheimer's—for reasons not yet known. The tangles, he feels, "are likely to be a better surrogate for tracking Alzheimer's progression and determining the efficacy of any given drug." These new imaging tools, he adds, "may work for related diseases that also have tangles, such as frontotemporal dementia, and could be used to assess tau pathology in the brain after a traumatic brain injury."

Diet and Exercise

We'll continue stressing the importance of a healthy diet, and of vigorous, daily exercise. Just in the last couple of years, researchers have found proof that especially with early-stage patients, the right diet and exercise not only block progression of the disease but enlarge the brain, grow new cells, and turn on various genes and proteins that keep brain cells alive. Other so-called lifestyle factors include moderate (or no) alcohol consumption and management of hypertension, high cholesterol, and diabetes.

Getting the Word Out to African Americans

We want *all* Americans to be aware of Alzheimer's symptoms, and to act on them if they appear. But we feel a special obligation to our fellow African Americans, given the shockingly higher incidence of Alzheimer's in the black community. We know that type 2 diabetes runs rampant in the community, too, and that there appears to be some link between the two diseases. Is it a coincidence that both of B.'s parents, along with all her father's siblings, and one of her three brothers, died of diabetes, and that B. then got early-onset Alzheimer's? I think it's all too likely that both of B.'s parents and her brother Gary, had they lived longer, might have gotten Alzheimer's and died of it instead.

All over this country, but especially in the South, African Americans are struggling with both early- and late-onset Alzheimer's, and not doing what they can do to save or prolong their lives. Not going to primary care doctors for candid talk about symptoms. Not getting PET imaging diagnoses. Not participating in clinical trials that can unlock the mystery of why twice as many African Americans as Caucasians get Alzheimer's in the first place—and which drugs, at which dosages, may at last be able to treat or even cure the disease in the black community. Tuskegee remains a horrible stain on the federal government and the scientists who administered it. But it's a long-ago time and place, and laws have been passed to keep it from happening ever again. Researchers have to tell you what they're giving you, how it might help, and what its side effects might be. And they have to get your consent.

I'll tell you this: I'm going out to help recruit participants for those trials. I can't make new drugs and I don't have the money to fund scientists to do it for me. But I do have a voice—a pretty loud one, I'm told—and I can use it to put out the word. It's very simple: you're either in one of those trials or you're not. You're part of the solution, or part of the problem.

Along this journey, I've learned to lower my expectations. I know some years may pass before a first generation of "disease-modifying" drugs—not just drugs that treat mild symptoms—gets to market and starts to change the story we know about Alzheimer's and its stages. I know, most important, that the chances of seeing the fog lift from B.'s brain are very slim. Yet in recent months, as I've talked to experts and learned more about this disease, two names have come up again and again: two researchers racing down similar paths to a possible breakthrough after all. As it happens, they work a short walk away from each other, in the research complex of Massachusetts General Hospital, overlooking the Charles River in Boston.

The drugs they're working with aren't new, exactly. What's new is their approach.

If they're right—and a lot of their colleagues think they are—the key to Alzheimer's may lie as much in when the right drug is given as in what it is.

THIRTY-TWO

BOSTON

Fall 2014–Winter 2015

D r. Reisa Sperling is a woman about half my size, all smiles and bustling energy. She's both a neurology professor at Harvard Medical School and director of Alzheimer's research at Boston's Brigham and Women's Hospital. In other words, she's serious. She's also full of hope for what she calls her A4 study.

Strictly speaking, the drug that Dr. Sperling is testing has already failed. It's called solanezumab—let's call it S-bub for short. The big pharmaceutical company Eli Lilly hoped it would block the forming of amyloid plaques. It didn't, so it failed its trial. But while S-bub didn't work on patients who actually had Alzheimer's, it did seem to help patients at an earlier stage: those who had signs of amyloid buildup but no cognitive impairment as yet.

Maybe the drug wasn't the problem. Maybe the timing was the issue.

For what she hopes will be the largest Alzheimer's prevention trial in the country, Dr. Sperling aims to have at least one thousand participants, spread over sixty sites. Each participant will be between sixty-five and seventy-five years old. Each must have two copies of the APOE-e4 gene—one from each parent—but no symptoms yet of Alzheimer's. Half the group will get S-bub; half will get a placebo. Sperling will track both groups for three and a half years.

Testing a drug for *prevention* of Alzheimer's is novel enough. But there's another twist to the A4 study I find especially intriguing. Sperling wants 20 percent of her one thousand participants to be African Americans. So does the National Institutes of Health, which is providing most of the A4 study's funding: $36 million. So far, unfortunately, Dr. Sperling has only fifty volunteers overall; of those, only six are African American. Here we are again: same old story. How are we going to learn why African Americans are twice as apt to get Alzheimer's if none of them will join the A4 study?

Dr. Sperling is doing all she can, visiting black churches, community centers, and more, to get out the word and line up participants. But she's starting to feel pressure to start on the trial with the fifty or so participants she has. She won't say where the pressure's coming from, exactly, but it's a fact that Lilly is now in a race with another company called Biogen that just won approval to start its own Phase III trial for an almost identical drug.

A five-minute walk from Dr. Sperling's office is a scientist who may be about to learn exactly how Alzheimer's works, and in the process give the world a whole new perspective on it, one that may make Alzheimer's as easy to treat as high cholesterol.

The first thing you notice about Dr. Rudolph Tanzi is his

intensity. He grins as he takes your hand; then he's off and running, rattling off medical jargon with a Boston accent as flat and heavy as any Kennedy's. At fifty-six, he's head of Massachusetts General Hospital's Genetics and Aging Research Unit, and teaches at Harvard Medical School. The hospital has taken over the old Charlestown Navy Yard and spiffed it up, but kept the red brick façade. Dr. Tanzi's office has a curving, brick-framed window overlooking the Charles River, and a desk dominated by three oversize computer screens, where the answers to Alzheimer's may lie.

Scientists may argue over who the leading figure in Alzheimer's research is, but nearly all put Dr. Rudy Tanzi in the top three. In the mid-1980s, he was one of the discoverers of the first Alzheimer's-related gene, APP (amyloid precursor protein), eventually known by those three variants APOE-e2, e3, and e4. In the mid-1990s, he helped find two more. Now he may be on the verge of his greatest discovery yet.

Dr. Tanzi is excited but cautious: he's been at this rodeo before. Back in 2001, when he published his book *Decoding Darkness,* about his early gene searches, he and his team were focused on three new drug trials, all trying to block amyloid plaques. All those trials eventually failed, as one after another of those drugs proved toxic in the human brain.

With that, the whole question of whether amyloid plaques cause Alzheimer's seemed up for grabs. Maybe it was the tau tangles after all. But in the ongoing debate—amyloid plaques or tau tangles?—Dr. Tanzi remained stubborn. He still felt the plaques were to blame.

On his way to a breakthrough in 2014 that would drastically

affect the debate, Dr. Tanzi saw his profile rise in ways he'd never expected. *GQ* magazine included him in a photo shoot called "Rock Stars of Science," paired with Aerosmith guitarist Joe Perry. When Dr. Tanzi told the rock legend he'd played organ in bar bands through his twenties, Perry suggested they jam. Dr. Tanzi ended up playing organ tracks on Aerosmith's next album. (Another *GQ* rock star of science was our own Dr. Sam Gandy of Mount Sinai.) A chance meeting led to a book collaboration with Deepak Chopra, the mind-and-body expert. *Super Brain* has since sold one million copies and spun off a PBS series hosted by Dr. Tanzi. But none of this took him away from what he calls his obsessive, almost pathological quest to crack Alzheimer's.

PET imaging was the key. With it, for the first time, scientists could see how early plaques began to form in people who would eventually get the disease. "We could see that amyloid begins in the brain fifteen to twenty years before symptoms," Tanzi explained. "By the time you show symptoms, amyloid growth is already plateauing." Maybe trying to treat the symptoms once they were pronounced was a fool's errand. "Giving a patient a drug for amyloid is like giving a patient who just had a heart attack some Lipitor," Dr. Tanzi declared. "You have to give it a lot earlier than that."

That was the epiphany that led Eli Lilly to retry S-bub on pre-Alzheimer's patients with amyloid plaques: the A4 study that Dr. Sperling is leading. It's the epiphany that has since led Biogen to come up with a similar drug. Both use antibodies that may block amyloid.

Last October, as these two drug prospects were squaring

off, startling news came from Dr. Tanzi's lab. Not another new drug to rival those two. Something bigger. A new tool to transform the field and test dozens, hundreds, thousands of possible Alzheimer's drugs, not over a period of years, but weeks.

"For the first time, and to the astonishment of many of their colleagues," the *New York Times* reported of Dr. Tanzi and neuroscience partner Doo Yeon Kim, "researchers created what they call 'Alzheimer's in a Dish'—a petri dish with human brain cells that develop the telltale structures of Alzheimer's disease." Tanzi and Kim had done it with human embryonic stem cells, growing them as neurons, then giving them Alzheimer's genes. Over time, the genes acted just as they did in human brains: creating amyloid plaques and tau tangles.

The implications are staggering. Until now, scientists have been forced to test possible new drugs one at a time in mice. Though genetically close to humans, mice are different enough that success with a new drug in mouse models is merely a good indication, not proof, that the drug will work in humans. That's one reason why Alzheimer's drug trials have so often failed. Worse, mouse trials take up to eighteen months.

Now that whole paradigm has been turned on its little mouse head. "So instead of waiting a year and a half with a mouse, we can test all twelve hundred approved FDA drugs and about five thousand Phase I safety trial drugs," Dr. Tanzi told me triumphantly. Drugs, that is, for any and all needs. "You don't know what might work with Alzheimer's. Who knows how many unexpected combinations we might get that work against it?"

At the same time, Dr. Tanzi's "Alzheimer's in a Dish" trick appears to transform, after thirty years, the great debate over whether Alzheimer's is caused by amyloid plaques or tau tangles. The answer is . . . plaques! Or to put it more conservatively: you don't get Alzheimer's *without* plaques. Just as Dr. Tanzi thought all along. "We get plaques in six weeks," he says of his petri dish stem cells, "then get tangles. If you stop the plaques, you don't get the tangles." So tau tangles aren't the sole cause of Alzheimer's, as some scientists believed. And they don't seem capable of causing Alzheimer's without plaques in the picture somehow.

But while this mechanism may be true in the "petri dish," when the cells are given the abnormal amyloid gene, the debate isn't quite settled. Howard Fillit, for one, continues to believe there are many causes of neuronal cell injury in the aging brain, with many of them, such as inflammation, oxidation, energetics failure, neuroprotection, and others being worthwhile drug targets, and beta-amyloid being one among them in the vicious cycle of neuronal injury.

Reisa Sperling has her own doubts, not so much about the science of Dr. Tanzi's petri dish breakthrough as about how much it matters in regard to getting new drugs to market. Reisa has boundless admiration for what Rudy Tanzi has contributed to the field, but ultimately, she says, it's about the trials. What works in a petri dish still has to be tested on human beings, and the ways in which new drugs interact with human biology— over a year, or two, or three—can't be predicted. In most cases, they can't be controlled, either. So again, what seems like the beginning of the end of the struggle to stop Alzheimer's is more like the beginning of the beginning. It's a better place to be than you were before, but you've still got a ways to go.

Whether it's game, set, and match or merely game, Dr. Tanzi has clearly made a profound contribution to Alzheimer's research. To him, it's part of the new big picture—and so are those mild-stage antibody drugs that Eli Lilly and Biogen are testing in people who have plaques and tangles, but not yet any symptoms of Alzheimer's.

"Here's my dream," Dr. Tanzi told me, leaning in as if to confide a secret. "Biogen's antibody opens the door to the notion of a statin for Alzheimer's." Statins, of course, are for lowering serum cholesterol levels to clear arteries and reduce the chance of cardiovascular disease. When Dr. Tanzi talks of a statin for Alzheimer's, he means a drug that works in the same way a statin for heart disease does. "Instead of measuring cholesterol, it's measuring amyloid," Dr. Tanzi said with an impish grin. "Instead of a blood test, it's PET imaging."

Dr. Tanzi sees a time, not far in the future, when a doctor looks at the PET amyloid image of a forty-year-old's brain and says, "You have way too much amyloid for a forty-year-old; you need to take a moderator like Biogen's."

Maybe it's a little white pill like Lipitor, Dr. Tanzi added, that can bring your amyloid down like Lipitor brings down cholesterol. So a doctor treats you before you have cognitive issues. "Remember these words," Dr. Tanzi told me: *gamma secretase modulator.*

That's the enzyme that will keep those amyloid plaques from forming, Tanzi explains, without doing any damage in the process—and keep a forty-year-old from getting the disease in twenty or thirty years.

.   .   .

Last night, B. and I curled up at home to watch the Oscars. Most of it was so boring that you could have Alzheimer's and not miss a thing. But toward the end of the broadcast, we perked up as the nominees for Best Actress were named. One was Julianne Moore, for her heartbreaking performance in *Still Alice* as a fifty-year-old dealing with early-onset Alzheimer's. I had taken B. to see the movie, and she'd loved it, even as it provoked a lot of tears. The envelope was opened, the card pulled out—and wow! Julianne Moore won! More surprising was what happened next. B. whooped with delight, pumped her fist, and cried, "You go, girl!"

Even now, we have moments like that.

Both of us, I think, have accepted that B.'s illness will only get worse. Those new drugs from Eli Lilly and Biogen, those breakthroughs in Boston, the new focus on prevention—we're simply too late for that, and we know it. I do have every confidence that in my lifetime, Alzheimer's will no longer be the all-powerful enemy that it is today. It will be, as the doctors put it, a managed disease, probably a treatable disease, maybe even a reversible disease. You just can't have 15 million Americans walking around in a fog, wandering off into the night. The drug companies *will* come up with a host of new drugs for the reasons they always do: public need and corporate profit. There *will* be answers. And fortunes will be made.

I'm hopeful—confident—that all this will come to pass. It's just hard right now to feel too happy. As I write these words, I'm at the dining table, looking out over the bay, and B. is on the living room sofa, fiddling with a word game she no longer knows how to play. Barring a miracle, those medical breakthroughs won't come in time to save a woman who has moderate-to-severe Alzheimer's, a woman who for twenty-two years has been my beloved wife.

I feel her over there, sitting quietly, waiting again for me to tell her what to do. I think what we'll do is get Bishop, and head down to the beach for a long winter walk, before the last of the daylight is gone.

LESSONS LEARNED

The Brain Registry

The easiest way to make a difference with Alzheimer's is to sign up to participate in a brain study trial. It helps to be sixty or over, but you certainly don't need to have Alzheimer's—or even worry that you might!—to participate. Brain-healthy participants are just as important as those who aren't: healthy "control" groups are an essential part of most trials, especially research trials, in which participants are simply observed over time.

Living in a major metropolitan area helps—that's where the medical centers are, and where research and drug trials for Alzheimer's are apt to be found. But there's another way to join, no matter where you live, and now I'm talking black or white, with or without Alzheimer's. It's called the Brain Registry.

Back at that Alzheimer's benefit luncheon, I met Dr. Michael Weiner, an internist and medical scientist who'd often worked over the years with our doctor, Howard Fillit. Dr. Weiner saw that with Alzheimer's research, the lack of trial participants was a stumbling block. "It's the biggest problem," he explained to me. "The high cost and difficulty of getting people into studies. Recruiting people, identifying them, screening them—it's a very messy, slow process. Most researchers still interview ten people for each one they get."

The other problem, Dr. Weiner saw, was that every study recruited for itself. "If two investigators in San Francisco are both doing neuroscience research, they will each have their own research teams and clinical trials and recruit participants individually. It's crazy!"

This year, Dr. Weiner created the Brain Registry, a website to enlist trial participants across the country. The trials are for various diseases, but Alzheimer's is one of them. All it takes is being eighteen or older and committing three hours a year to cognitive testing. As scientists come up with new drugs to test on Alzheimer's, they'll need participants—and now they may find them through the Brain Registry, instead of putting ads in college newspapers or on Craigslist.

After just six months in operation, the Brain Registry has signed up ten thousand candidates already. To date, most of those are in the San Francisco Bay Area, because that's where Dr. Weiner lives and works. But this is just the start. "Our goal is to go global," he told me. "And all the data that comes from those trials will be shared with anyone who might benefit from it. Clinical data, that is: a participant's personal data is fiercely guarded."

Go for it! Visit www.brainhealthregistry.org.

A NASTY LITTLE SECRET

Some months ago, I found myself scanning the obituaries with an interest I'd never had before. Oh, sure, I read the obits of people I'd heard of or known. But I didn't go down the day's list of paid obits in the *New York Times,* looking for how each person had died. Now I did—and what I found, to my surprise, is that almost no one died of Alzheimer's. I guess in a way I was looking for comfort in numbers—or maybe it was misery in search of company. I didn't find it. And why was that, with

Alzheimer's the sixth-highest cause of death in the country—or even the third, depending on which organization is doing the counting?

The fact, as Dr. Fillit explained, is that many of those people *had* died of Alzheimer's; it just wasn't listed as the cause of death. Strictly speaking, it was the indirect cause. And a lot of grieving families preferred to list, as the cause of death, the final complication that Alzheimer's led to: a stroke, heart attack, or pneumonia.

Pneumonia is the most common of those end-stage courses. By then, a patient is immobile, which affects his lungs' capacity to expand and manage secretions properly. That leaves him susceptible to infections, including pneumonia. An inability to swallow may allow foods, liquids, and saliva to enter his airways, increasing the odds of pneumonia. In fact, as many as two-thirds of the people who die from Alzheimer's are listed, in their obits, as dying from pneumonia. Or complications from pneumonia. Or just "a long illness."

The hospitals are partly—maybe mostly—to blame. They're being too literal in listing pneumonia as the cause of death. Technically they may be right, but with Alzheimer's, pneumonia is merely the grace note. Or as that grim saying has it, the old man's friend, since it's relatively painless and the patient dies in bed.

The hospital may list pneumonia to be medically exact, but the family knows better. Any family whose loved one has just died of Alzheimer's *can* request that Alzheimer's be listed in an obituary as the cause of death, but all too few do. Some families may just be too grief-stricken to think about this, but let's be blunt: a lot of families stick with the hospital's listed cause of death to avoid the still-strong stigma of Alzheimer's, both on behalf of their just-deceased loved one—and themselves.

I say the hell with that.

You want to see Alzheimer's get more federal funding? You want to keep a next generation from suffering as much with this awful disease as your family has? Then do the right thing: insist that Alzheimer's be listed as the cause of death. Change comes with numbers. Political change, I mean. Dr. Fillit is sure that far more Americans have Alzheimer's right now than the 5.2 million estimated by the Alzheimer's Association. He thinks the real number is 10 million, maybe more. Where are those other five million? Hiding in their houses—or being hidden— their illness dismissed as routine aging, their deaths recorded as anything but Alzheimer's. The bigger the real number of Alzheimer's patients, the bigger the real number of Alzheimer's deaths, the more our government will be pushed into giving it the funding it deserves—as the third-biggest killer in our country.

When it comes, don't be embarrassed to list the true cause of death for your loved ones. That, along with signing up with the Brain Registry, may be the most significant move you can make to help manage, and ultimately stop, this disease.

The Spiritual Side

For better or worse—well, let's just call it worse—spirituality has played no real part in B.'s adult life or mine. B. remembers those door-to-door days selling *The Watchtower* as if they were last week, but neither her father's faith as a Jehovah's Witness nor her mother's as a Baptist left much imprint on her. As for me, I've just never felt the need to enter a church. Even in us, though, Alzheimer's has stirred something that feels close to spiritual.

It starts with questions. Why do any of us have to suffer this terrible disease, knowing that our minds and memories are being dulled and destroyed one by one? What God could possibly let our brains and bodies disintegrate in this way? If there is a God, and if he does allow this kind of suffering, what message might he be trying to send? Is the point, perhaps, for all of us to appreciate, more keenly, what life we have left? Is it about living in the moment—truly in the moment, the way only a person with Alzheimer's can?

Lately, I've been doing some reading on this. You wouldn't believe how many technical papers there are out there on spirituality and Alzheimer's. As if scientists could measure spirituality like blood pressure! One theme that comes up a lot is how helpful religious faith is for people with mild-stage Alzheimer's. Not only does it ease their anxiety: it seems to slow their cognitive decline. For a boy from Bed-Stuy who never saw much point in church, that's a very persuasive reason to start going. The Alzheimer's Foundation of America's website notes three academic papers that all reached the same conclusion: regular attendance at church kept participants' minds sharper. Maybe it was praying, especially prayers known from childhood—and hymn singing, too. That kind of weekly joining in on long-familiar words and music might stimulate the temporal lobes, the scientists suggested, or increase memory-strengthening chemicals in the brain. Being involved with a church and its congregations, the scientists added, might ease anxiety. It might also provide comfort and hope. The scientists stopped short of proselytizing, but did point out that hundreds of studies had shown that religious individuals cope better with stress and depression.

Googling around, I found one academic paper with just the title I wanted: "Using Spirituality to Cope with Early-Stage Alzheimer's Disease." Of course B. was now a bit past the early stage, but I still identify the two of us as dealing with early-stage Alzheimer's: a little lingering denial, I guess. In any case, this paper, from a team at Vanderbilt University, suggested that spirituality in *any* manifestation has a beneficial effect. Some of the trial participants defined their spiritual world as nature, others as a pragmatic, guiding principle in their lives, still others as the explanation for suffering and setbacks. Some, to be sure, also associated spirituality with God and churchgoing. But I was gratified to think that a belief in God wasn't the only ticket you could punch to get the physical and psychological benefits of spirituality.

Sometimes now, B. and I talk about life and what it means, what's important and what we can do to get the most from what remains. I'd like to think that in the next years, we'll do more talking like this.

One comforting thought is that even as B. continues to change, she's still the same person I married, twenty-two short years ago. Which is to say that even as Alzheimer's diminishes her mind, and periods of anger and depression increase, the essence of who she is—her soul—remains the same.

For now, remarkably, B. still looks as beautiful as she ever was. Not only that: she's fit enough to walk the length of Manhattan in red spike heels! The moments of dislocation and dysfunction are increasing, the inability to follow what's said, or to do tasks that take multiple steps—all this points in the obvious, inevitable way. For now, though, she's still more B. than not.

When those changes do occur, I hope that I'll be able to do what I'm hoping you can do, too: not lose sight of the soul within. Keep communicating with the soul you know and love, even if she grows immobile and seems not to react. Studies have shown that patients with end-stage Alzheimer's do hear, think, and feel, even if they seem to have vanished from the ruined bodies they inhabit. I know I'll be right there, holding the hand of the woman I love. I guess that's spirituality, too, of the human spiritual kind.

Good luck to us all.

ASSOCIATIONS AND ORGANIZATIONS

Abe's Garden
Alzheimer's and Memory Care Center of Excellence
115 Woodmont Blvd.
Nashville, TN 37205
www.abesgarden.org
Email: Use the "Contact Us" form on their website.
Phone: (615) 345-9575
Abe's Garden is a nonprofit partner with the Vanderbilt Center for Quality Aging, at Vanderbilt University in Nashville, Tennessee, to provide a national best practices model of residential living and adult care programs for those affected by Alzheimer's disease and dementia. The goal is to provide unparalleled respite care and residential living for individuals with Alzheimer's or dementia and to become a center of knowledge for individuals with the disease. Abe's Garden also seeks to improve the lives of affected families, and professional care partners.

Alzheimer's Association
225 North Michigan Avenue
17th Floor
Chicago, IL 60601-7633

http://www.alz.org
Email: info@alz.org
24-hour/day hotline: (800) 272-3900
Phone: (312) 335-8700

The Alzheimer's Association, or Alz.org, as it's also known, is the big enchilada: the world's leading nonprofit health organization for Alzheimer's care, support, and research, working globally but also locally.

Alz.org is, in fact, the largest nonprofit funder of Alzheimer's research, and has played a role in most of the last three decades' advances. Since 1982, it has awarded more than $315 million in grants to more than 2,200 scientists. It publishes a scientific journal, *Alzheimer's & Dementia,* and maintains an international society to keep researchers up to date. It also holds an annual international conference.

Alz.org is just as committed to enhancing care for individual patients and their caregivers. Its Alzheimer's and Dementia Caregiver Center (http://www.alz.org/care/) provides comprehensive online resources and information. Alz.org also administers twenty thousand education programs and communicates caregiving information in fifteen languages. It helps patients find clinical trials through its service TrialMatch (http://www.alz.org/research/clinical_trials/find_clinical_trials_trialmatch.asp). It also provides search assistance for patients who wander, through its safety services, Comfort Zone and MedicAlert + Alzheimer's Association Safe Return. www.alz.org.

**Alzheimer's Disease Education and Referral Center
(ADEAR Center)**
National Institute on Aging
US Department of Health and Human Services
Building 31, Room 5C27
31 Center Drive, MSC 2292
Bethesda, MD 20892
www.nia.nih.gov/Alzheimers
Email: adear@nia.nih.gov
Phone: (800) 438-4380

A US government institution established in 1990 to "compile, archive, and disseminate information concerning Alzheimer's disease" for health professionals, people with Alzheimer's and their families, and the public. The ADEAR Center is a service of the National Institute on Aging, which conducts and supports research about health issues for older people, and is the primary federal agency for Alzheimer's disease research. The ADEAR Center strives to be a current, comprehensive, unbiased source of information about Alzheimer's disease.

Alzheimer's Drug Discovery Foundation
57 West 57th Street, Suite 904
New York, NY 10019
www.AlzDiscovery.org
Phone: (212) 901-8000

This nonprofit drug research foundation, started by brothers Leonard and Ronald Lauder of the Estée Lauder family, is dedicated to rapidly accelerating the discovery and development of new drugs for Alzheimer's disease. Nearly 100 percent of contributions go directly to Alzheimer's drug research, which the ADDF funds through a venture philanthropy program. The ADDF has provided over $70 million to more than 450 drug research programs in a score of countries. The founding executive director and chief science officer of the ADDF is Howard Fillit, MD, a leading neuroscientist and geriatrician who specializes in the diagnosis and care of people with Alzheimer's disease, including B. Smith, in his limited private practice.

Alzheimer's Foundation of America
322 Eighth Avenue, 7th Floor
New York, NY 10001
www.alzfdn.org
Email: Use the "Contact Us" form on their website.
Phone: (866) 232-8484 (Toll Free) or (646) 638-1542

The Alzheimer's Foundation of America (AFA) strives "to provide optimal care and services to individuals confronting dementia, and to their caregivers and families—through member organizations dedicated to improving quality of life." AFA unites more than 1,700 member organizations from coast to coast that are dedicated to meeting the educational, social, emotional, and practical needs of individuals with Alzheimer's disease and related illnesses, and their caregivers and families. Under AFA's umbrella, these organizations collaborate on education, resources, best practices, and advocacy.

The Cure Alzheimer's Fund

www.curealz.org

The Cure Alzheimer's Fund is a nonprofit organization founded in 2004 by three families who were frustrated by the slow pace of research. Leveraging their experience in venture capital and corporate start-ups, the founders (Henry McCance, Phyllis Rappaport, and Jacqui and Jeff Morby) came together to build a new venture-based Alzheimer's research fund designed to dramatically accelerate research. Dr. Rudolph Tanzi is the fund's Research Consortium chair.

Geoffrey Beene Foundation—Alzheimer's Initiative

1101 K Street NW
Suite 400
Washington, DC 20005
Email: alzheimers@geoffreybeene.com
http://geoffreybeene.com/Alzheimers-initiative/

The Initiative is a nonprofit organization underwritten by the Geoffrey Beene Foundation that is committed to providing catalyst funding to innovative new projects that advance awareness, diagnosis, and research on the early stages of Alzheimer's disease.

BOOKS

To date, Alzheimer's has inspired a mostly grassroots response in terms of books that address its many issues. Some of the best yet written are:

Slow Dancing with a Stranger: Lost and Found in the Age of Alzheimer's, Meryl Comer; HarperCollins, 2014.
The 36-Hour Day: A Family Guide to Caring for People Who Have Alzheimer's Disease, Related Dementias, and Memory

Loss, 5th edition, Nancy L. Mace and Peter V. Rabins; Johns
    Hopkins University Press, 2011.
*Surviving Alzheimer's: Practical Tips and Soul-Saving Wisdom
    for Caregivers,* 2nd edition, Paula Spencer Scott; Eve-Birch
    Media, 2014.
*Chicken Soup for the Soul—Living with Alzheimer's and Other
    Dementias—101 Stories of Caregiving, Coping, and Com-
    passion,* Amy Newmark and Angela Timashenka Geiger;
    Chicken Soup for the Soul Publishing, 2014.
*The Emotional Survival Guide for Caregivers: Looking After Your-
    self and Your Family While Helping an Aging Parent,* Barry
    Jacobs; Guilford Press, 2006.
*Alzheimer's Disease and Other Dementias: The Caregiver's Com-
    plete Survival Guide,* Nataly Rubinstein; Two Harbors Press,
    2011.
*Learning to Speak Alzheimer's: A Groundbreaking Approach for
    Everyone Dealing with the Disease,* Joanne Koenig Coste;
    Mariner Books, Houghton Mifflin, 2004.
*A Caregiver's Guide to Alzheimer's Disease: 300 Tips for Mak-
    ing Life Easier,* various authors; Demos Medical Publishing,
    2006.
*Creating Moments of Joy for the Person with Alzheimer's or De-
    mentia: A Journal for Caregivers,* 4th edition, Jolene Brackey;
    Purdue University Press, 2008.
On Pluto: Inside the Mind of Alzheimer's, Greg O'Brien; Codfish
    Press, 2014.

AIDS AND TOOLS

Alzheimer's Awareness Purple Bracelet
From the Alzheimer's Association. Features the association logo and
the message "reason to hope." http://www.amazon.com/Alzheimers
-Awareness-Purple-Silicone-Bracelet/dp/B0058E4G2Q/ref=sr_1_20?ie
=UTF8&qid=1418660291&sr=8-20&keywords=Alzheimers.

Alzheimer's Navigator

A service of the Alzheimer's Association. This online tool helps patients and family members create a customized Alzheimer's Action Plan. https://www.Alzheimersnavigator.org/?_ga=1.52378607.735698444 .1418131901.

Dementia Digital Calendar Day Clock

A digital clock designed for people with early-stage Alzheimer's or memory loss that displays the exact time in a large, bright, and clear display that can be easily seen from across the room. No abbreviations are used, so no memory is required. Sold by GeriGuard Solutions. http:// www.geriguard.com/DayClox-p/dcx-800.htm.

Home Safety for Patients with Alzheimer's Disease

Brochure put out by the National Institute on Aging in August 2010. Available at http://www.nia.nih.gov/Alzheimers/publication/home -safety-people-Alzheimers-disease/introduction.

iTrack

The iTrack, designed by ElectroFlip, is a GPS tracking device for finding patients. The device uses cellular and GPS technology and is designed to be used in conjunction with cell towers and GPS satellite. According to the manufacturer, it is easier to use than a cell phone and all you need to operate it is a prepaid SIM card. The iTrack uses up to thirty-two satellite channels and cellular towers for accuracy within ten feet. It comes equipped with long-life dual lithium-ion batteries that last up to six days on a single charge. http://itrack.electroflip.com/index.html.

ON THE HORIZON

Marco Polo

An application for iPhones or Android devices that prompts the patient with compromised memory with words or phrases that might be useful, based on daily routines. In development by the Technologies for Aging Gracefully Lab (TAGlab). http://taglab.utoronto.ca.

MemeXerciser

MemeXerciser will allow a person to wear "pervasive lifelogging systems" that have cameras, audio recorders, location trackers (much like a GPS system), and other technologies embedded in them. Without being prompted, these technologies will record experiences and events for the user. This helps the person with impaired memory be able to confidently recollect recent experiences, and reduces the burden on caregivers as well. http://www.cmu.edu/qolt/Foundry/documents/memexerciser_factsheet.pdf.

Comic Relief

Even now, with B. in Stage Five, we find a lot to laugh about. I would say not a day goes by without us cracking up about something, whether it's Bishop, our wacky Italian mastiff, or something we see on TV. Also, almost every night, we watch comedies—either movies or television shows. With B. living more and more in the moment, I think humor brings her intensified pleasure. When she's laughing, she can't be depressed; my own sense is that laughter, for a moment at least, obliterates the challenging reality of her life and makes her truly happy. Anyway, you can hardly lose for trying, right? So here, for the heck of it, is a grab bag list of B.'s and my favorite comedies:

Television: *Modern Family*—the "mockumentary" on ABC that chronicles three families living in Los Angeles and struggling to master the ever-more-complex business of parenting. B. laughs so hard at it she starts to weep.

Cedric the Entertainer in anything and everything he's done, from *Who Wants to Be a Millionaire* on television to his many movie comedies, from *Top Five* and *Planes: Fire and Rescue* to *Johnson Family Vacation* and *Big Momma's House.*

Movies: *As Good as It Gets* (1997), with Jack Nicholson, Helen Hunt, Greg Kinnear, and Cuba Gooding Jr. Grumpy and misanthropic Nicholson is drawn into the lives of his favorite waitress and a gay neighbor.

Clueless (1995)—Alicia Silverstone, Paul Rudd, and more: hilarious, sharp-edged look at Beverly Hills teenagers. Later a television show.

Dumb and Dumber (1994)—Jeff Daniels and Jim Carrey drive across the country to Aspen, Colorado, to return a briefcase whose contents they never question: in fact, the case contains ransom money. Okay, this one really *is* dumb. But like I said at the start: no matter how corny, tasteless, or silly, if it makes you laugh, go for it.

Harvey (1950)—And finally, a blast from the past: Jimmy Stewart as an alcoholic whose friend is a six-foot invisible rabbit. Redone as a television series in 1998.

ACKNOWLEDGMENTS

Every story that needs to be told starts in the heart of the storyteller—but goes no further without someone else who believes in that story as well. To our friend and agent Barry Weiner, your belief in B. and me, and in the rightness of making our story public, made this book possible. It simply wouldn't exist without you.

To Janis Donnaud, the literary agent whom we originally met at a friend's Christmas party, we heard early on about your expertise and class, and are grateful we got to experience them firsthand. You make your writers' work sharper and more focused, and our book is the better for that.

To our editor Heather Jackson, who embodies caring and thoughtfulness, we thank you for encouraging us to write honestly and personally about a subject many still shy away from—but one that must be discussed. We love who you are and what you represent.

To Dr. Sam Gandy, a doctor with a down-home approach and a scientist's yearning for unlocking the code that will eventually bring about the demise of Alzheimer's, we thank you. To Dr. Martin Goldstein, a guy with the gentlest bedside manner, and the gift for translating medical jargon into language we could understand, thank you for doing all you've done for B. and me.

Dr. Howard Fillit is a person we've come to call a good friend. Whenever and wherever he was, we could reach out, and he would be in touch in the blink of an eye. We are so grateful to have a doctor and scientist who treats us like an old-style family practitioner, and who somehow finds the time to head up the Alzheimer's Drug Discovery Foundation, funding so many promising drugs and therapies.

The title of this book is *Before I Forget,* but the people above are people we always want to remember. And we will always remember Michael Shnayerson, a writer with kind eyes and a quick wit; above all, an absorber of human experience. His craft is writing, his gift is storytelling, but his true value is in being a good friend.

And to our daughter, Dana Carlisle. From the moment I looked in your eyes at birth, you have been a joy. From the moment B. took you under her wing, you have lifted her up as she did you. We couldn't have written this book without your keen observations and unflagging honesty. Along the way, you have taught me as a caregiver how to be more patient, more understanding, and more resilient in the face of something that truly no one can prepare for. We love you, we cherish you, we are thankful for you.

To Lois Smith, a sister-in-law who has always been Barbara's sister, thank you for rounding out B.'s story. To Cynthia Badie-Beard, you and Barbara always say you're pretend sisters, but I know that's just a ruse to throw people off, for the love you have between each other only true sisters could share.

And finally, my wife.

I always wanted to have someone in my life who represented an ideal but might not be obtainable. You are that ideal, and I am so grateful for the honor and pleasure of your company, and for the privilege of sharing your life. Most of all I am forever thankful for your eyes that look upon me with love, and for that smile that has captured my heart and millions of others. We all know the secret to you, B.; it's very simple: what we see in you is what we get—the real deal.

INDEX

ABOUT THE AUTHORS

B. SMITH

B. Smith is a multi-media pioneer in the lifestyle and entertaining realm: the first African American woman to become a national arbiter of taste, with an audience that cut across all racial and ethnic lines. Born in Everson, Pennsylvania, she began her career as a top fashion model for the Wilhelmina Agency, becoming the first black face on the cover of *Mademoiselle* and appearing on numerous covers of *Essence* and *Ebony*, among other national publications. She also represented major brands, from Crest to Pillsbury to Betty Crocker. In the mid-1980s, she opened her first eponymous restaurant in New York's theater district; in its appeal to both black and white patrons, including many celebrities, it broke color barriers, too. B. Smith went on to write three books on entertaining: *B. Smith Rituals and Celebrations*, *B. Smith's Entertaining and Cooking for Friends*, and *B. Smith Cooks Southern Style*. Frequent appearances on national television shows like *Good Morning America* led to her own nationally syndicated television show, *B. Smith with Style,* which ran profitably for eight years and set another precedent:

the first-ever nationally syndicated lifestyle show by an African American. A national magazine, *B. Smith Style*, was also launched at this time. Along with their New York restaurant, B. and her husband, Dan, oversaw two others, in Washington, D.C., and Sag Harbor, New York, where they now live full-time.

DAN GASBY

Dan Gasby, B.'s husband for twenty-three years, is also her business partner in all her ventures. Raised in the Bedford-Stuyvesant section of Brooklyn, New York, he made his way through Colgate University and became a television sales and marketing executive. Eventually he created the syndicated television show *Big Break with Natalie Cole,* a precursor of *American Idol,* which ran in over 180 markets and launched the careers of R. Kelly and Eric Benet. After meeting B. in the late 1980s, he built her multi-talented presence into a national brand, overseeing all her ventures. Along with caretaking B., he is now involved with several start-ups in digital media.

MICHAEL SHNAYERSON

Michael Shnayerson is a longtime contributing editor to *Vanity Fair* and the author or coauthor of six books, among them *My Song,* the bestselling memoir by legendary entertainer and civil-rights activist Harry Belafonte. Most recently, he published *The Contender* (Twelve), an unauthorized biography of New York governor Andrew Cuomo.